Society
and Health

An introduction
to social science
for health professionals

Edited by

Graham Moon
and Rosemary Gillespie

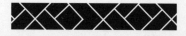

First published 1995
by Routledge
11 New Fetter Lane, London EC4P 4EE

Simultaneously published in the USA and
Canada
by Routledge
29 West 35th Street, New York,
NY 10001

Text design: Barker/Hilsdon

Typeset in Janson Text and Futura by
Florencetype, Stoodleigh, Devon

Printed and bound in Great Britain by
Biddles Ltd, Guildford and King's Lynn

*British Library Cataloguing in Publication
Data*

A catalogue record for this book is
available from the British Library

*Library of Congress Cataloguing in
Publication Data*

A catalogue record for this book has been
requested

ISBN 0-415-11021-1 (hbk)
ISBN 0-415-11022-X (pbk)

Society and Health

Society and Health: An introduction to social science for health professionals examines the ways in which sociocultural factors affect health care practice. Health care professionals do not simply supply the treatments that illness or injury demands. They must make informed decisions guided by economic, sociological and legislative constraints. The book also examines how external factors impact on individual health and attitudes to health care. For example, specific health issues can be easily linked to the home or work environment, whilst a patient/client decision about when, where and even if to seek treatment may be linked to considerations of finance or location.

The contributors have drawn on their wide-ranging experience of teaching health professionals to demonstrate the scope and application of social science concepts and theories to health and health care. Part one provides the unfamiliar reader with a contextual framework for health and modern health care. Part two looks at people's encounters with ill health and the interaction between patients/clients and the health services. The final part examines the National Health Service, its inception, development and position today, focusing specifically on the implications of recent policy changes.

A social scientific approach encourages health professionals and those in training to take account of the sociocultural influences governing themselves, the institutions they represent and their patients. Thinking critically about these matters creates the potential for improving health and health care.

Graham Moon has fifteen years' experience as a teacher and researcher of health issues. He was involved in the integration of Nurse Education into the curriculum at the University of Portsmouth, where he is Professor of Health Services Research.

Rosemary Gillespie was formerly a Senior Ward Sister and Nurse Teacher and is now Senior Lecturer at the University of Portsmouth.

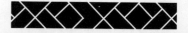

LONDON AND NEW YORK

Contents

v

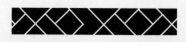

Illustrations

Figures

Tables

Contributors

Chloe Gerhardt is a freelance writer. She formerly taught medical sociology and undertook consultancy work in a variety of health care settings. Her health-related interests focus on development and health and critiques of biomedicine.

Martin Giddey has had considerable experience of the NHS as a clinical, professional manager and educator. He is currently Senior Lecturer in Social Policy in the School of Social and Historical Studies, University of Portsmouth and has special interests in health policy, mental health and community care.

Rosemary Gillespie is a Senior Lecturer in Health Studies in the School of Social and Historical Studies, University of Portsmouth. She has a background in nursing and a major involvement in teaching social science to health professionals. Her research interests focus on the sociology of health and illness and the sociology of the body.

Ian Kendall is Principal Lecturer in the School of Social and Historical Studies, University of Portsmouth. He has long-standing research interests in health and social policy with a particular interest in welfare history.

Graham Moon is Principal Lecturer in the School of Social and Historical Studies, University of Portsmouth. He was centrally involved in the initial development of the University's Project 2000 nurse education course and has worked in health services management. His research interests are in health geography, quantitative health planning and the medico-legal interface.

Nancy North is Senior Lecturer in Health Studies in the School of Social and Historical Studies, University of Portsmouth. Her main interests are in health policy and, in particular, in health commissioning. She spent 15 years working in the NHS.

Susan Phillips is Lecturer in Medical Sociology in the School of Social and Historical Studies, University of Portsmouth. She is a sociologist with research interests in doctor–patient communication.

Robin Prior is Principal Lecturer in the School of Social and Historical Studies, University of Portsmouth. His interests focus on information technology and its application in the social sciences.

Acknowledgements

We would like to thank our colleagues for their contributions to this text. They have produced their chapters (generally) on time and have acquiesced gracefully to our editing. We would also like to thank the various groups of health professionals who have participated in our classes over the past few years and have been the test bed for the ideas brought together in this book. Finally we would like to thank our families whose tolerance, as ever, has been remarkable.

Introduction

- Graham Moon
- Rosemary Gillespie

Social science and health

This book is about the application of social science concepts to health and health care. Social science is of central importance in understanding both the individual and the society in which they live. It also helps us to look critically at some of the things that we frequently take for granted, for example, the family, social roles, social inequalities and the determinants of good health. In the context of this book, social science is used to look critically at some 'taken-for-granted' assumptions about health, illness, disease and medical care. Is good health, for example, something that is in our own hands, determined by the choices we make, or is it determined by social forces? Is medicine scientific, objective, rational and always the best option available or does it, at times, operate in the interests of certain groups, such as the health professionals who provide the service, or organisations associated with, and supportive of, health care, for example, the drugs and medical technology industries? Rarely will a 'correct' answer be found within social science, rather,

1

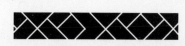

a range of interpretations and perspectives will be demonstrated. Social science sometimes even questions the very existence of objective knowledge or reality.

The term 'health' is generally understood as something to which we all aspire, an objective reality that individuals either have, or do not have. The reality, however, is far more complex, and health is difficult both to define and measure. The World Health Organization (WHO) defined health in 1948 as 'not merely the absence of disease and infirmity but complete physical, mental and social wellbeing'. It is therefore not simply the opposite of being sick; it is about 'wellness' in its fullest social and spiritual sense. Illness and disease are also complex issues. Illness is generally assumed to be the subjective experience of feeling unwell, whilst disease is associated with the clinical malfunctioning of the body.

An understanding of what constitutes good health or being ill may vary from one individual to another and it may change during a lifetime with ageing. Developing a disease may change a person's understanding of what constitutes good health, and the way they relate to their body; poor health may never go away, but often can be minimised through diet, exercise or pain control. Concepts of health, illness and disease change in accordance with changing ways in which society perceives health. Cartesian philosophy led to an understanding of the body as a machine, made up of a series of parts, many of which were destined to fail, or go wrong, during a person's lifetime. Modern society views the body more *holistically* – taking account of the whole environment in which the body is situated.

Health, disease and illness are therefore, as well as being highly subjective phenomena in their own right, also affected by a multitude of individual and social factors. They will reflect a person's occupation, whether they have a job, their income, the levels of stress they experience, the lifestyle they lead, the choices they make, and the amount of pollution present in their environment or workplace. They will be associated with social structures, for example, social class, or other social groupings that a person belongs to, such as gender and ethnicity.

Health care can also be understood in a social science context. Using a health care service or working in a health care setting involves social transactions between different types of health professionals and between health professionals and patients/clients.

These transactions take place in situations which are closely affected by changing health policy; they are constrained by political decisions about resources, service management and service innovation.

Organisation

This text has been designed to be a concise introduction to the central issues concerning health and health care in contemporary British society. It is written primarily for an audience of health professionals undergoing basic training. It draws on the contributors' experience of teaching social science to a range of health professionals. The key aim is to convey the scope and utility of a basic range of social science concepts and theories.

Part one is intended to contextualise health and health care within the social, historical, geographical and demographical framework within which the service is delivered. Chapter 1 assesses the key processes of demographic and epidemiological transition in order to demonstrate the influences which have brought about our current population structure. Chapter 2 explores the ways in which the family and community are inextricably linked with health and caring. It focuses on the ways in which social change has significant implications for the ways in which much health care is delivered and maintained. Chapter 3 offers an historical analysis of the development of the dominant biomedical view of health care in Britain. Chapter 4 examines the critics of this approach to care. They have argued that medicine may not always be as rational, altruistic and objective as it has been assumed. Chapter 5 explores the social model of health, and highlights the ways in which the social sciences have attempted to provide a useful framework for the understanding of health, illness, disease and disability.

Part two develops a sociological analysis of the ways in which individuals and groups respond to the experience of illness and disease. It also considers the ways in which they come to seek help for their problems from a variety of agencies, which may or may not include the health care services. Chapter 6 focuses on the social and cultural factors that underpin people's understanding of health and illness, and the processes involved in seeking care. This will enable health professionals to understand the experiences of people in their care. It should also enable them to communicate more effectively and ultimately provide better care. Chapter 7 examines the interaction that takes place between health care professional and patient/client both at the individual level and in relation to social groups. Clinical interaction is of the utmost importance to the delivery of care and can have significant implications for both the communication that takes place between health care professionals and patients/clients, and the outcome of care. Chapter 8 considers the problems associated with health care institutions. It also examines the nature of professional power in relation to health care work.

Part three considers the social, economic and political implications of current health policies in the UK. We currently live during a time of great uncertainty and change in service provision; this section of the book is important for understanding the dynamics of these changes and their implications for the health professional. Chapter 9 considers the political history of the British National Health Service and Chapter 10 provides an analysis of the most recent reforms. Chapter 11 outlines the major changes in NHS management during the 1980s and the impact on patients and professional groups. Chapter 12 explores the evidence and explanations for inequalities in health in British society. Chapter 13 evaluates the increasing importance of economics in the delivery of health care and explores the ways in which decisions made by managers and clinicians are based on limited resources which constitute considerable challenges to those responsible for providing care. Chapter 14 evaluates the importance of inter-agency collaboration in a service where patients are spending increasingly shorter periods of time in hospital, requiring the support of a variety of different groups and agencies, increasingly drawn from voluntary and commercial agencies.

How to use the book

The organisation of the book is set out in a logical order that will enable the reader to build upon material that has gone before.

The reader will gain the greatest understanding of the application of social science to the study of health, illness and disease from reading the entire book in the sequence in which it is presented. However, we have also taken care to ensure that the book can be used flexibly, with the reader dipping into each chapter, which constitutes a self-contained unit, making use of cross-referencing to other chapters where appropriate.

Each chapter opens with a summary of the main themes to be covered in the chapter. This summary can be referred to afterwards to make sure that those themes have been assimilated, and to facilitate revision. At the end of each chapter exercises and activities are included to enable the reader to reflect, consolidate and share knowledge, and apply it to relevant practice. Further reading is identified, as an introductory text can never hope to do more than offer a brief insight into what are often complex and interesting debates.

Finally, as an extra revision aid, key terms and concepts are highlighted in the index in bold type, directing the reader to the page on which the definition or meaning of the term is given in the text.

Part one

Health
and health care
in context

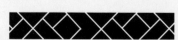

Chapter 1

Demographic and epidemiological change

- Graham Moon

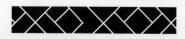

CONTENT

- Demographic indicators

- The demographic transition

- Epidemiological indicators

- The epidemiological transition

- Geography and health

AIM

The chapter will provide a historical overview of the interrelationship between health and demographic, social, economic and cultural trends.

G OOD HEALTH IS A FUNDAMENTAL GOAL for people and the societies in which they live. Individuals hope for a life free from illness and pain, and societies, through the acts of governments, promote policies designed to counteract ill health. As the introduction to this book showed, the meaning of the word health is hotly debated. These debates will be revisited in Chapter 5, but see p. 81 the present chapter will take a simplistic view of health, linking it to disease and death. This simplistic perspective will be used to introduce some of the key concepts used in the study of 'health'; it will also underpin a review, which will continue into the next chapter, of the 'health' status of the British population. The intention in the present chapter is to assess broad processes of *demographic* and *epidemiological* change over long periods of time. This 'long view' will demonstrate that many of the key facets of present-day health status are derived from processes that have been in operation for some time. The next chapter will consider some of the more recent factors which influence health status.

KEY TERMS

Demography

The study of populations and population change. Usually associated with a focus on birth, marriage and death.

Epidemiology

The study of the patterns and determinants of disease distributions in populations. Includes both death and sickness.

Vital statistics

In Britain today health status is relatively high. In comparison with the past, things have improved greatly. Comparisons with some less-developed countries also indicate that the people of Britain enjoy a relatively satisfactory health status. Yet neither of these comparisons is wholly satisfactory. There are diseases prevalent among the British population today which were of little importance even as recently as a hundred years ago, for example, both AIDS and sudden infant death syndrome (SIDS) have only been recently recognised. Similarly, while Britain may have a broadly satisfactory health status in comparison to other countries, it does not compare well with its partners in the European Union (EU). Table 1.1 shows some *vital statistics*, or key indicators of life, which summarise important variations between the countries of the EU.

Although this chapter will be more concerned with historical comparisons, the indicators in Table 1.1 will be used to develop an understanding of some key concepts in the measurement of health status. The indicators in Table 1.1 are generally felt to be key indicators of a country's overall health status. They are used by bodies such as the Organization for Economic Co-operation and Development (OECD) and the World Health Organization (WHO) to gauge the success of health care programmes and the level of health development.

Life expectancy refers to the average length of life which an individual can expect, counting from the day they are born. It is usually calculated separately for men and women and can also be recalculated to provide life-expectancy figures at particular ages. Thus, the standard life expectancy at birth in Britain can be subsetted to provide a figure of 73 for men and 79 for women; the higher figure for women is replicated in most countries. Life-expectancy figures can also be recalculated to show how many more years of life a person of a particular age might expect. Not unexpectedly this assessment of the average remaining years of life decreases as a person ages. However, it also varies from place to place and between men and women.

The *infant mortality rate* (IMR) is generally felt to be an extremely sensitive indicator of overall health status. Not only can it be argued to reflect the relative stress which a nation places on the health care of its very young population – the future of the

TABLE 1.1   European Union: key health indicators (1990)

Country	Life expectancy	Infant mortality rate	Crude death rate	Birth rate
Belgium	m72.0 w78.9	8.4	10.6	12.0
Denmark	m72.6 w78.2	7.5	11.9	12.4
France	m73.4 w81.8	7.2	9.2	13.3
Germany	m72.0 w78.1	7.5	11.5	11.2
Greece	m74.6 w79.8	9.7	9.2	10.1
Ireland	m72.0 w77.7	8.2	8.9	14.9
Italy	m73.6 w80.4	8.6	10.1	10.0
Luxembourg	m71.8 w79.2	7.3	9.9	13.0
Netherlands	m73.9 w80.3	6.5	8.6	13.2
Portugal	m69.8 w77.3	9.8	9.7	11.0
Spain	m73.4 w80.5	7.7	8.5	10.2
United Kingdom	m73.3 w78.8	7.4	11.3	13.8

Source: World Health Statistics Annual

country – it also reveals much about variations in factors such as maternal nutrition, social care and the provision of child welfare. The calculation of the IMR is a relatively straightforward matter: the number of children aged under 1 year who die in any particular year is divided by the number of children born alive in that year and then multiplied by 1,000. Nevertheless, the IMR is often subdivided to identify other more specific measures: stillbirth, perinatal mortality and neonatal mortality rates. These reflect the relatively greater risks faced by newborn children and the specific risks faced in the period just before birth.

KEY TERMS

Stillbirth rate

Number of stillbirths (foetal death between the 24th week of pregnancy and the due-date of birth) divided by the total number of live and stillbirths. Usually expressed per 1,000 total births per year.

Perinatal mortality rate

The number of stillbirths plus the number of deaths in the first week of life in a given area during a given time divided by the total number of live and stillbirths. Usually expressed per 1,000 total births per year.

Neonatal mortality rate

The number of deaths in the first 28 days of life in a given area during a given time divided by the total number of live births. Usually expressed per 1,000 live births per year.

Trends in death rates may also be calculated relatively easily. The *crude death rate* (CDR) is simply the number of deaths in a given year divided by the total population. This measure is, however, not particularly helpful. It considers all deaths throughout the age span, yet it is known that the chances of dying are much greater for very young and very old people. The crude death rate also considers men and women together, yet it was shown earlier in this chapter that women live longer than men. In sum, in a population with more men and an older age structure, the crude death rate is likely to be raised in comparison with a younger population with a greater proportion of women (Jones and Moon 1987: 52–4). As a consequence, there is a need to standardise the measurement of death to take account of the age and sex structure of the population. The *standardised mortality ratio* is the most commonly accepted outcome of standardisation. This is calculated using the procedure set out in Box 1.1 and allows a much better comparison of mortality statistics.

BOX 1.1

Calculating a standardised mortality ratio

Age	Population of study area A	Reference death rate[1] B	Expected deaths A × B
<1	0.74	19.78	15
1–4	2.93	0.76	2
5–14	8.38	0.40	3
15–24	8.83	0.92	8
25–44	13.41	1.62	22
45–64	18.36	13.45	247
65–74	8.23	51.82	426
>75	4.64	137.42	638
Total			1361

Actual deaths: 1223

SMR = (1223/1361)(100) = 90

Properties: SMR > 100: mortality worse than average
SMR = 100: average mortality
SMR < 100: mortality better than average

Note: (1) a reference population for a country might be world standard set of death rates; for a town in a country it will normally be the national death rates.

Finally, consideration can be given to the *birth rate*. This provides a measure of the rate at which a population would increase if population increase only involved births. It is calculated by dividing the number of live births in an area during a specific time period by the estimated population of the area. The time period chosen is normally one calendar year and the rate is generally expressed per 1,000 persons.

An allied measure, which also allows a focus on the reproduction of the population, is the *fertility rate*. This is a rather more complex measure which divides the number of live births in an area during a specific time period by the female population of child-bearing age in that area. Child-bearing age is, by convention, defined as 15 to 44 years. Again, this rate is expressed per 1,000 women.

The demographic transition

If data were to be collected for any one country in Table 1.1 for the years prior to, say, 1990, an interesting pattern would emerge if enough data were collected. Over a time period of perhaps 300 years, there would be clear evidence of a phenomenon known as the *demographic transition* (Figure 1.1). This concept can conveniently be separated into four stages (Meade *et al.* 1988):

1 High stable: Both birth rates and death rates are relatively constant, fluctuating at high levels.

2 Early transition: While birth rates are maintained at a high level, death rates commence a period of steady year-on-year reduction.

3 Late transition: The reduction in death rates begins to slow and, at the same time, a steady reduction in the birth rate occurs.

4 Low stable: Both birth rates and death rates regain relative stability but at much lower levels in comparison to stage 1.

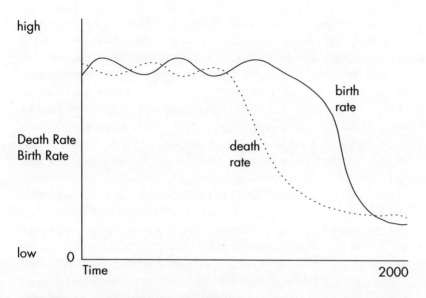

FIGURE 1.1   Demographic transition

By the simple interaction of its two key components, the birth rate and the death rate, the demographic transition demonstrates, at a basic level, some of the dynamics underlying population change. During the high stable phase, new births will simply function to replace the dying. As both the death and the birth rates are similar there will be little or no population growth. Furthermore, the effect of the high death rate and the high birth rate will be to limit the numbers of older people and raise the numbers of younger people. As the transition phases are entered, so population growth takes place. A societal need to ensure the reproduction of the population ensures that the high birth rate is maintained after the death rate begins to fall. The consequence of this is a rapid natural increase in the population which levels off as the birth rate, too, begins to fall. During the later stages of transition, there is a falling birth rate and a stable death rate. This means that infants no longer enter the population cohort in great quantity. Consequently, the population begins to age and, eventually, the low stable stage is reached when there are substantial numbers of elderly people in the population and, again, little or no population growth.

Of course, birth and death rates are not the only components of population change. Emigration and immigration are equally important in determining the age structure of a population. Nevertheless, the demographic transition gives some useful insights which can be extended by considering linked processes of social change. First, while the high stable stage will be characterised by large families as a consequence of high birth rates, transition is associated with a move to smaller families. Second, as the process happens through time, the transition also reflects the impacts of such factors as the changing role of women, the uptake and improvement of birth control methods and improvements in medicine, nutrition and hygiene. Third, the key factor in the demographic transition is the infant survival rate. As more infants survive to adulthood, so the death rate becomes associated more clearly with old age. Much of the fall in the death rate through the period of transition is, in fact, a consequence of improvements in infant survival. Indeed, once account has been taken of improvements in infant mortality rates, life expectancy has changed little in over one hundred years.

The full four-stage demographic transition which has been discussed so far is, naturally, an idealisation. Reality is never quite so simple – the transition provides a *model* or general framework against which we can compare 'real-world' situations and which we can use as the basis for the development and testing of ideas. Most industrialised countries are well advanced through the transition and provide exemplification of the low stable phase; in some, birth rates will even have fallen below death rates. However, non-industrialised, rural and, particularly, less-developed countries may exhibit the characteristics of earlier phases in the transition. Cultural factors may militate against reductions in the birth rate, economic and political factors may cause raised death rates as a reflection of poverty, famine, war, environmental degradation and poor availability of health care. The starting positions of each country will also, of course, be different. It is therefore hardly surprising that no one country conforms exactly to the model of the demographic transition.

Epidemiological indicators

Death rates and standardised mortality ratios cannot only be calculated for overall death statistics but also for individual causes of death. Identifying these individual causes and their relative importance allows a more detailed knowledge of the health of the population to develop. Each cause of death will raise questions about the process and management of the disease, the lifestyle of the deceased and the environment in which he/she lived. Thus, deaths from different cancers may variously raise questions about working in the nuclear power industry, smoking and the availability of screening services.

The categorisation of causes of death has a long and complex history (Nissel 1987: Chapters 9 and 10). In Britain, some cities published, albeit irregularly, 'Bills of Mortality' in the sixteenth century. These were somewhat haphazard in their categorisation, reflecting, to an extent, the imperfect nature of medical knowledge at the time. In 1836 an amendment to the Births and Deaths Registration Bill brought about *civil registration* of death and the process of agreeing names for all fatal conditions began. Central to this quest was William Farr, at the time Statistical Superintendent at the General Record Office and therefore responsible for official statistics. He circulated a categorisation to all medical practitioners in 1845 and requested its use to avoid ambiguity. In 1853 Farr liaised with a Swiss statistician D'Espigne to produce an internationally agreed categorisation. This was not, initially, widely used, but eventually it came to form the *International Classification of Diseases* (ICD).

The ICD was adopted in the United Kingdom in 1911 and was adapted in 1948 for use in the study of morbidity (illness) as well as mortality. It is now the responsibility of the World Health Organization (WHO), a Geneva-based international organisation. Periodic revisions ensure that the classification remains up to date with contemporary medical knowledge and the use of the tenth revision has just commenced. The ICD classifies deaths according to the location within the body where the cause of death was situated. Thus, malignant neoplasms (cancers) may be linked to particular sites, such as the pancreas, and even to parts of sites, such as the head of the pancreas.

Such epidemiological detail originates ultimately from death certificates completed by medical practitioners who use their knowledge to indicate the disease or condition leading directly to the death. Other significant conditions, contributing to, but not actually causing death may also be noted. This allows a distinction to be drawn between the prime cause of death and other conditions present at the time of death – it also allows for an understanding of the constellation of multiple causes which are, nowadays, typically present when a person dies. The information is converted from a written statement to an ICD code by workers at the Office of Population Censuses and Surveys (OPCS) using standard WHO manuals. The data are then checked and stored on computer for subsequent publication and analysis.

Needless to say, the ICD suffers limitations. Long-term analysis of changes in the incidence of deaths from certain causes may be hindered by changes in the coding framework between revisions of the ICD. Diagnoses of the cause(s) of death may be also inaccurate: Alderson (1983: 21) suggests that major inaccuracies may characterise up to 5 per cent of certified causes of death. Finally, the ICD, despite attempts to make it comprehensive, is also, undeniably, most effective in the analysis of mortality. Its use in morbidity studies is limited – most morbidity involves no contact with health practitioners and, consequently, recording of the episode of ill health does not take place. Even when contact with health professionals does occur, the mechanisms for effective storage of cause of death information and conversion to ICD coding may be absent. Only in the case of people hospitalised with acute health problems will there be likely to be an even marginally satisfactory ICD record of morbidity.

The ICD is particularly limited when it comes to the epidemiological study of mental health and learning difficulties. In a sense the classification medicalises these matters, an approach which may be unacceptable to many practitioners in both fields. ICD codes are available for both learning difficulties and mental health problems. They are, however, little used and practitioners have developed systems of classification which are more appropriate. In the mental health area, one such classification is the *Diagnostic and Statistical Manual* (revision three) (DSM III).

Notwithstanding these problems and shortcomings, it is still possible to compile powerful and interesting analyses of the current epidemiological situation using cause-of-death information. As the next chapter will show, in Britain today by far the most important causes of death are circulatory diseases (heart attacks, strokes) and cancers. The position differs little between men and women. As with vital statistics, it is possible to extend an analysis back in time to see how this position has come about.

The epidemiological transition

Circulatory diseases and cancers are examples of what are known as *degenerative* or *chronic* diseases. These chronic diseases have not always been the major causes of mortality and morbidity in the British population. Nor is chronic disease, in a worldwide sense, always the major cause of present-day mortality and morbidity in every country. Attention needs also to be given to the role of a second category of diseases: *infectious diseases* (Box 1.2). In Britain these were once of prime importance in generating mortality. In some countries they remain the key killers. The process of shifting from a situation characterised by infectious disease to one typified by chronic disease is known as the *epidemiological* or *mortality transition* (Omran 1971).

BOX 1.2

Some chronic and infectious diseases

Chronic diseases	Infectious diseases
Ischaemic heart disease	Bubonic plague
Diabetes	Measles
Cerebro-vascular disease (stroke)	Pertussis (whooping cough)
	Yellow fever
Arthritis	AIDS
Rheumatism	Malaria
Cancers	Cholera
	Typhoid

A simplistic presentation of the epidemiological transition would see it as a linear progress from a situation dominated by infectious disease to one dominated by chronic disease (Figure 1.2).

This model might, as with the demographic transition, proceed conceptually through four stages:

1 Age of epidemics: Levels of infectious disease are very high; all age groups are affected but particularly children. Consequently, life expectancy is low and infant mortality is high.

2 Receding epidemics: Infectious diseases are controlled and become progressively less important as causes of mortality. In particular young people escape infectious disease mortality.

3 Age of chronic disease: Chronic disease becomes the main cause of death. Life expectancy rises, infant mortality is low.

4 Delayed degenerative disease: Further rises occur in life expectancy but quality of life may not improve as extreme old age becomes characterised by multiple health problems, including mental health problems and untreatable but non-fatal chronic disease.

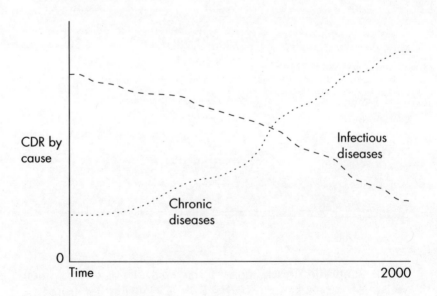

FIGURE 1.2 Epidemiological transition

In Britain some 250 years ago life was short and often unpleasant, certainly for people outside the wealthier echelons of society. Every fifth baby would die before it was one and few people lived beyond thirty. This situation was, if anything, made worse by the rapid industrialisation and urbanisation of the country in the subsequent 100 years. Conditions of extremely bad sanitation, poor housing and general overcrowding contributed to making a situation where infectious disease could and did flourish. Not only did coughs and sneezes spread disease, so too did dirty water, damp housing and poor waste disposal. Very young children were particularly vulnerable to the many infectious diseases which were always present (*endemic*) as well as the regular *epidemics* of rarer diseases which spread rapidly through the population.

The epidemiological transition in Britain and other 'developed' countries was, in many ways, about a shift of mortality from young to old people. As such it can be linked with the demographic transition and the centrality of infant survival to the falling death rate. The mortality toll of industrialisation and urbanisation, not only on the very young, but also on the potentially productive workers in the economy, was recognised by *sanitary reformers* of the mid-nineteenth century (see Chapter 3) and attempts were made to address the worst evils of poor hygiene and bad housing. Children were among those to benefit from these reforms. Although many examples of insanitary living remained, the impact of bad hygiene was reduced and the ability of this vulnerable section of the population to survive was raised. see p. 57

Two other factors also assisted infant survival. First, by the mid-nineteenth century, as will again be seen in Chapter 3, *medicine began to gain in effectiveness*. A biomedical understanding of disease processes enabled treatments for infectious diseases to be developed. By the mid-twentieth century vaccination programmes were in place for many of the formerly fatal infectious diseases. These programmes were, and remain, primarily targeted on children. Second, as will be seen in Chapter 9, policy developments were also extended beyond hygiene – embryonic attempts were made to make health care available to a wider public than those able to afford to pay for the services of a *personal doctor*. Among the first to benefit from these measures were children. see pp. 56–7

see pp. 150–52

As a consequence of sanitary reform, biomedical advance and social policy developments, by the end of the second phase of the epidemiological transition, infectious disease had been effectively superseded as the major killer. It will hopefully be clear from the weight of discussion in the previous two paragraphs that there is a clear consensus that the key factor bringing about this epidemiological transition was sanitary reform (McKeown 1979, 1988). Many of the medical advances happened substantially after the sanitary reforms had begun to clear away the conditions which allowed infectious disease to flourish. Figure 1.3 illustrates a key example. It remains a topic of considerable debate however as to which strategy – sanitary, medical or social – is most effective in phases three and four of the transition. What is clear, however, is that the later phases of the transition place mortality firmly as a problem of older age groups and indicate that the health experience may increasingly be one of complex multiple chronic morbidities interacting together to reduce the quality of life.

While it is generally agreed (McKeown 1988; Chen *et al.* 1992) that the epidemiological transition is now well advanced in 'developed' countries, it must, of course, also be remembered that, like the demographic transition, it is a model. It cannot be universally applied everywhere and 'read-off' as an expected outcome of universal processes. In Britain it took perhaps 200 years to run from phase one to phase four. In some countries the process was accelerated as major government action and economic success brought a rapid defeat of infectious disease. In others, initial successes were followed by problems, such as war, famine or economic disaster, which have delayed the unfolding of the transition, leaving countries suffering heavily from both infectious and chronic diseases. Some countries, of course, notably in Africa, continue to experience conditions reminiscent of the first stage of the transition. Nor is it impossible for the transition to be reversed and Frenk *et al.* (1989) note that different groups within societies may proceed more or less rapidly through the transition. As Jones and Moon (1992) argue, the transition is a complex and potentially useful tool. It should not be used in an overly simplistic sense nor should it be assumed that it provides a complete description of a process which is undoubtedly continuing.

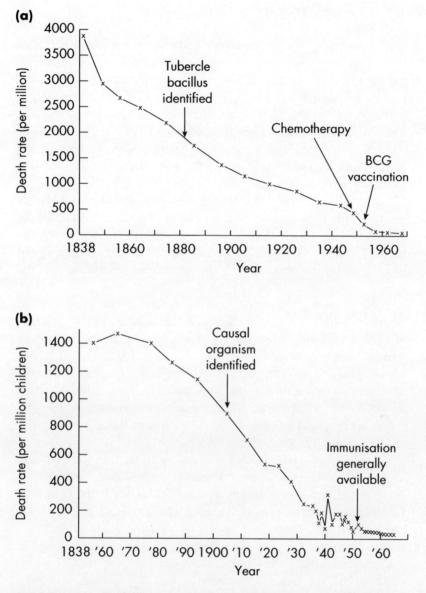

FIGURE 1.3 Declining mortality from tuberculosis and whooping cough: the effect of medical intervention (a) respiratory tuberculosis: mean annual death rates (b) whooping cough: death rates for children aged under 15. *Source*: McKeown (1979)

Health and geography

In the context of the demographic and the epidemiological transitions Britain today is a relatively advantaged country in health terms. The death rate is relatively low and epidemic infectious disease is no longer a substantial problem. This is undoubtedly a happy situation, yet, as the preceding section has shown, it is not without its problems. A high life expectancy is likely to be accompanied by multiple health problems. These health problems along with others, including not inconsiderable levels of infectious disease, are also, as was suggested earlier and as will be seen in Chapter 12, unequally distributed between different population groups. This final section of this present chapter will look briefly at the way in which they are additionally distributed unequally between places. This short consideration of the geography of ill health will, in common with the rest of the chapter, take a historical view.

In pre-industrial times a broad picture of the geography of health would portray, for the general population, a situation of almost uniform experience of generally poor health by today's standards. There would be localised areas of extreme ill health where famine or crop failure occurred. In keeping with the epidemiological transition, much of the ill health would be related to infectious disease and, when epidemics occurred, developing urban areas would exhibit the highest rates as the diseases spread rapidly among the denser populations.

The rapid industrialisation and urbanisation of the late eighteenth and nineteenth centuries created, as has already been noted, markedly insanitary conditions in Britain's towns. Consequently, urban areas became characterised by markedly poorer mortality rates in comparison to rural areas. Two issues flowed from this. First, there emerged a vision of rural Britain as a wholesome and healthy place; the town was perceived as inherently unhealthy. Second, because urbanising Britain was geographically concentrated around industrial opportunities associated with coal, cloth, wool, trade and steel, a clear urban geography of ill health emerged with certain cities experiencing particularly poor mortality rates. The social and housing conditions of these towns and the conditions of life for their residents laid the basis for this ill health.

   The impact of the health-related consequences of industrialisation can be traced to the present day and is evident in the most
general sense in a marked north–south divide in health status
(Smith 1989: 32–8; Townsend *et al.* 1988a). More detailed
epidemiological studies confirm the existence of this geography
of ill health. Charlton *et al.* (1983) collected information on
'preventable' deaths – deaths which might not have occurred if

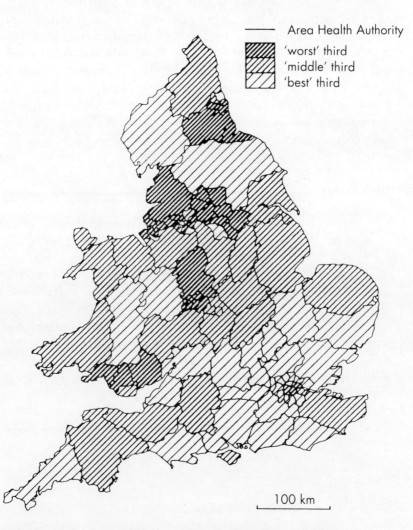

FIGURE 1.4   Geographical variation in conditions amenable to
medical intervention. *Source*: Charlton *et al.* (1983)

adequate medical care was given. For the period 1974–8, they identified twelve causes of death which varied significantly between areas and identified the worst and best areas on each indicator. They then created an overall measure and standardised for social conditions. The results were striking (Figure 1.4).

Recent evidence from the 1991 Census of Population indicates that morbidity also exhibits a clear geography. Data at the regional scale revealed that the proportions of residents with a self-reported illness were highest in Wales (16.4 per cent) and in Tyne and Wear (16.0 per cent). Within these regions the figures were highest in the South Wales valleys, Newcastle and Sunderland. Self-reported illness was lowest in the outer metropolitan area of South East England. These differences could only partly be explained by regional differences in age distributions – areas with the highest numbers of pensioners had lower-than-average rates of long-term illness.

CONCLUSION

This chapter has presented two models for understanding historical changes in demography and epidemiology: the demographic and the epidemiological transitions. An assessment has been made of the utility of these models in relation to Britain. It should be clear that the demographic and epidemiological situation today is very different from that of a hundred years ago. Although they remain important topics for a health professional, infant mortality and infectious disease are no longer the severe everyday problems they once were. Instead the health professional faces the problems of a growing elderly population: mental ill health and multiple chronic illness.

1 Review the material in this chapter and attempt to draw out the implications of each stage of the demographic and epidemiological transitions for the work of the health professional. You may wish to distinguish between the contemporary implications and the legacy today.

2 Assemble some evidence for geographical variations in mortality at a national and local scale. What factors do you think are behind these variations?

3 Try to construct a profile of the vital statistics for your home area. How do they compare to national statistics?

Guided Reading

This chapter endeavours to simplify some fairly complex arguments and debates. You should read the references to gain a fuller insight into the demographic and epidemiological transitions. You should also try to develop your knowledge of the general evolution of patterns of demographic and epidemiological change. The recommended references on the latter are Open University (1985a,b, 1993).

Chapter 2

Health, family and community

- Susan Phillips

- **Historical variation in family and community**

  – Demographic variation

  – The changing family

  – Sentiment, policy and the reality of community

- **Families, communities and care**

  – Who cares ?

  – The impact of informal care

AIM

The chapter will review conceptions of the family and ideas about community, drawing out the linkages with health.

T HE TERM 'HEALTH CARE' in modern western society often conjures up images of high-technology hospitals and health centres; images of nurses and doctors among many other uniformed professionals; and images of a modern medical regime incorporating pain-relieving and life-saving drugs and breath-taking surgical techniques. The fact that families and communities might be crucial and influential providers of care is sometimes underestimated (Oakley 1993). However, the majority of us grow up being cared for by a family of one kind or another with the consequence that family care is actually more normal than is generally realised.

see p. 57

The subject of this chapter is the relationship between family, community and health. The terms 'family' and 'community' need some clarification since neither are a hard or fast entity.

KEY TERMS

Family

Those to whom one is related and with whom one lives, or, in a broader sense, those to whom one is related but may not live with.

Community

Can be taken to include friends, neighbours, self-help groups, churches, community centres, interest groups and clubs. It carries with it a notion of geographical proximity.

The problem of deciding what counts as 'family' is one that arises later in this chapter in the discussion of the changing family and a dilemma also arises in deciding the proper role for families to play in the care of those who need short- or long-term care. It should become clear that the way we define 'family' has a partial impact on the role we expect it to play in the provision of care. Similar and related arguments apply to 'community'.

Social scientists have also commonly made a distinction between *formal* and *informal care*. This distinction is also by no means clear-cut since carers who fit into the formal category sometimes work in the community. GPs and district nurses are examples of these. Sometimes carers who fit into the informal category offer care through official or state organisations. Voluntary workers in hospitals are an example of these. The formal and informal sectors of care provision are interrelated and interdependent. It is, however, the informal provision of care with which we are primarily concerned in this chapter.

KEY TERMS

Nuclear family

A cohabiting unit of mother, father and their children. Usually contrasted with the extended family, an ever rarer phenomenon, in which the nuclear unit is extended by cousins and grandparents.

Throughout most of this chapter, reference is made predominantly to family rather than community. The reason for this is simply that the majority of informal care has been found to be provided by family members (Walker 1982). Community, however, remains an important part of the chapter. First, as will become clear, community impacts on family and vice versa. Second, and, perhaps, more importantly, 'community care' is the current preference in British health policy. The demands made on this form of care provision depend on numerous factors including the demographic characteristics of a population, the nature of families, and the nature of communities and attitudes towards the notion of community. The next section of this chapter is therefore devoted to discussing these factors. A third section of the chapter discusses the interaction of families, communities and care.

Family and community in contemporary Britain

A basic background to demographic change has been discussed in Chapter 1. Demographic variables relevant to family, community and health include how many people are born – the birth rate – and how many people die, in particular, the age at which people die. Rates of birth and death determine the age structure of any population and thereby influence potential demand for health care. As will become apparent, the age structure of a population also has an impact on the ability of a population to care for those in need.

see pp. 14–16

    Figure 2.1 illustrates clearly how the UK experienced a post-war 'baby boom' after the Second World War which persisted into the early 1970s. In 1951 the birth rate was 15.9 per 1,000 of population rising to a high of 18.8 in 1964. It then fell to 16.1 in 1971 and further to 11.7 in 1977. Between 1977 and 1991 it increased slightly and varied between 13 and 13.9. According to projections by the Office of Population and Census Surveys, it is likely to drop to between 12 and 13 between now and 2025.

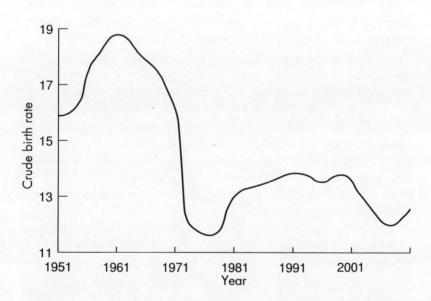

FIGURE 2.1 Crude birth rate: UK: 1951–2025 (actual and estimates). *Source: Social Trends,* HMSO, 1993

The result of the post-Second World War baby boom was high demand for maternity and child care services at the time of the baby boom. The subsequent result is a migrating population bulge (Giddens 1989). As those born during the baby boom grow up and mature to adulthood, so the population bulge ages. Consequently, the population bulge during the 1990s is constituted of adults born during the baby boom who are now approximately between 20 and 40 years of age. This translates to very high demand for adult-centred health care facilities, as illustrated later, and fierce competition for employment, education and training for adults.

It has been suggested that the population bulge represents a demographic time bomb set to explode when the population bulge reaches retirement age and, therefore, creates very high demand for old-age-related health and welfare services over and above that resulting from the general process of demographic transition. A question arises as to how this high demand for health and welfare services will be catered for. The balance between formal and informal provision of health care comes into question. Can the formal sector cater for increasing demand for care? Is the formal sector the most appropriate provider of care or is the informal sector – family and community – more able to provide a better quality, more appropriate or perhaps cheaper service?

The crude death rate (CDR) refers to the number of deaths see p. 14 per 1,000 population in a given time period. The CDR can be re-expressed as an age-specific death rate which refers to the number of deaths per 1,000 population in a specified age group. Table 2.1 clearly illustrates that the likelihood of death increases with age as would naturally be expected. The table also shows how deaths for all age groups dropped between 1961 and 1991. This also accords with expectation since the general standard of living has improved since 1961. What is significant is that the biggest drop in deaths occurred in age groups 60–79 years and 80+ years. In 1961 the death rate for ages 60–79 years was 49.15. This figure had dropped to 36.4 in 1991. This represents a drop of almost 13 deaths per 1,000 population aged 60–79 years between 1961 and 1991. For the age group 80+ years the death rate had dropped from 163.7 in 1961 to 132.8 in 1991 – a drop of almost 31 deaths per 1,000 population aged 80+. The drop in the death rate for younger age groups was less significant. For example, in the age group 15–39

TABLE 2.1 Changes in age-specific death rates: UK: 1961–91

Year	Age group					
	1–14	15–39	Females 40–59 Males 40–64	Females 60–79 Males 65–79	80+	All ages
1961	0.5	1.1	8.4	49.2	163.7	12
1971	0.5	0.9	8.1	43.7	153	11.6
1981	0.4	0.8	7.3	41.3	146.6	11.7
1991	0.3	0.8	5.3	36.4	132.8	11.3

Source: Social Trends, HMSO, 1993

years the rate dropped by approximately 0.3 per 1,000 population from 1.1 in 1961 to 0.8 in 1991.

What all these figures mean is that people are living significantly longer now than they did in 1961 and before, and that more people are living to be over 60 or even 80, 90 or 100 years of age. The consequence of a falling death rate for those aged 60 or over, coupled with a low and decreasing birth rate is that the UK increasingly has an ageing population. Partially as a result of this ageing population, there is now a very high demand for health care services in the UK. Figure 2.2 shows that self-reported long-standing illness increases gradually with age. In 1991 65 per cent of those aged 75 years and over reported long-standing illness compared to 41 per cent of those aged 45–64 years and 23 per cent of those aged 16–44 years.

Figure 2.3 illustrates that reported acute sickness according to days of restricted activity per person per year also increases with age. In 1991 those aged 16–44 years reported an average 17 days of restricted activity per year whilst the age group 45–64 reported an average of 29 days and the figure for those aged 75+ was 57. Furthermore, greater age correlates positively with average number of NHS GP consultations. In 1991 those aged 65+ visited NHS GPs on average six times per year compared to four times for those aged 16–44 years and three times for those aged 5–15 years (OPCS 1993).

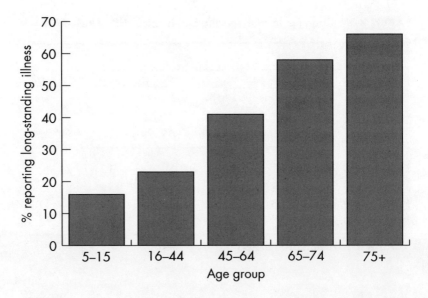

FIGURE 2.2   Self-reported long-standing illness by age: GB: 1991.
Source: General Household Survey, 1993

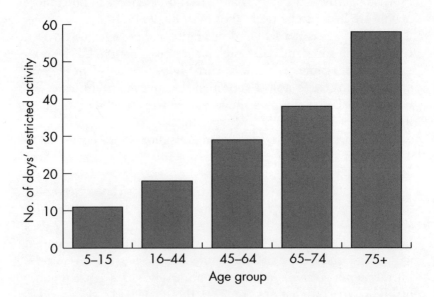

FIGURE 2.3   Acute sickness: average number of days of restricted activity per person per year: by age: GB 1991.
Source: General Household Survey, 1993

The linkage of an ageing population to a rising demand for health care has, in turn, resulted in rising health care costs. The problem of rising health care costs has become increasingly pertinent not only because of the demands made by an ageing population, but also as a consequence of the continuing development of modern high-technology medicine. Innovation and development in medicine has brought the possibility of treating more illnesses and therefore, more people. Demographically determined high demand for health care coupled with technologically determined high potential to provide that care has, during recent decades, raised questions, first, about how best to fund health care and secondly, how to provide the best quality and most appropriate care. Although government responses to these questions are set out in depth in later chapters, it is important in this present chapter to note that these responses have fundamentally been about the balance between formal and informal provision of care. The ability of the informal sector to provide care is centrally influenced by the nature of family (since family has been found to be the predominant provider of informal care).

The changing family

The nature of families influences the ability of families to provide care for those who need it. Families in Britain today exist in a wide variety of forms, just as they undoubtedly always have done. Despite this diversity it is possible to identify dominant family types and also to identify changes or trends in dominant family types over time. Unfortunately it is not possible to identify families that easily in official statistics; a surrogate indicator has to be used. Households are generally taken as synonymous with families which is not altogether satisfactory as some families may not live together as a household and some households will not be family units. This reveals an ongoing problem in the description and measurement of families in that families are not fixed or rigidly defined entities.

The bar graphs in Figure 2.4 illustrate how some types of household occurred less frequently in 1991 than in 1961. The household type which has decreased most significantly is that made up of a married couple with children – the *nuclear family*. In 1961 38 per cent of households were of this type. In 1991 this figure had dropped to 25 per cent. Household types which had increased most significantly in Britain were one-person households and single-parent families. In 1961 just 11 per cent of households consisted of a person living alone. This figure had risen dramatically to 27 per cent in 1991. Single-parent families had also increased significantly from 6 per cent in 1961 to 10 per cent of all households in 1991. These figures mean that more people are living alone in the 1990s than in the past, that more parents are finding themselves alone when bringing up children, that more children live with only one parent and that the family which is most often thought of as the norm or even the ideal type – the nuclear family – is becoming less common.

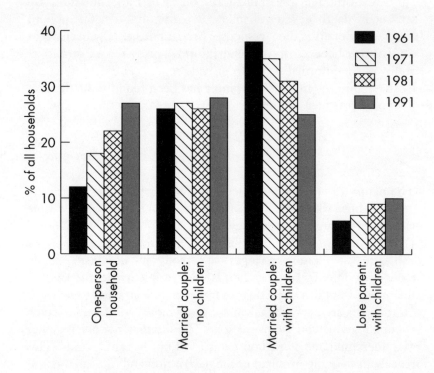

FIGURE 2.4 Changes in most common household type: GB: 1961–91. *Source: Social Trends*, HMSO, 1993

Formal care

That care provided by official or state organisations through such services as hospitals and health centres.

Informal care

That care provided by members of families or communities.

How can the changing size and structure of households be explained? Undoubtedly the demographic shift to an ageing population at least partly explains the dramatic rise in people living alone. Secondly, a high and rising divorce rate has contributed to the diminishing number of nuclear families and the increasing existence of single-parent families between 1961 and 1991. The divorce rate in England and Wales, referring to the number of people divorcing per 1,000 married, increased from 2.1 in 1961 to 12.9 in 1990 (HMSO 1993). Some changes in family composition are also due to a dramatic alteration in society's views of how families should be. In particular, birth outside marriage has become increasingly acceptable to the extent that live births outside marriage increased from 8.1 per cent of all live births in 1971 to 32.3 per cent in 1991 (HMSO 1993).

The changing nature of the family over time influences the ability of families to provide health care. Demographic change to an increasingly ageing population coupled with increasing numbers of people living alone and single-parent families raises questions about the viability of the family as a basis for care provision. These questions become more problematic when considered in the context of the changing nature of the wider community settings within which informal care is meant to take place.

Sentiment, reality and 'community'

The nature of a community obviously has an impact on the ability of that community to provide informal care for those in need.

Philip Abrams and colleagues (Snaith 1989), reporting on ten years of research into neighbourhood and social policy, find some discrepancy between sentiments and policy about community and what actually happens in the community. They report that the concept of 'community' is grounded in sentiments about creating a more caring society by transferring responsibility for caring from the public or state domain to the private or domestic domain:

> The myth of traditional community life as a densely woven world of informal strongly caring networks serves to prop up a belief in the possibility and desirability of renewing or reinvigorating laudable, traditional ways of helping people on a local basis.
>
> (Snaith 1989: 132)

The reality behind this myth was one in which the traditional, close-knit, caring community was a feature of a troubled past when close communities, by being the basis of care provision, effectively rendered life more pleasant than it otherwise would have been. The traditional community was a feature of a society where women stayed at home and where geographical mobility was limited. Although there were exceptions, many traditional communities were also characterised by homogeneous class structures and ethnic similarity.

In the past fifty years the characteristics which underpinned the traditional notion of community have rapidly disappeared. Urbanisation and redevelopment have contributed substantially to the process, not always with beneficial results. Society today is also characterised by a high geographical mobility as a consequence of which people seldom put down roots in a location for a long enough period for community ties to develop. Home-making women were central to traditional communities, yet now increasing numbers of women take full-time paid employment in a welcome challenge to gender inequalities. Finally, ethnic diversity has radically changed British society for the better.

Families, communities and care

Having considered some of the possible implications of demographic change, of the changing family, of economic circumstance and of the nature of community, it is now necessary to discuss two closely related topics: first, the extent to which families and communities have been empirically found to provide informal care and the way that this compares or contrasts to theory, and, second, the impact of informal caring on those who care informally and on those who receive it.

Who cares?

The empirical evidence concerning family, community and the provision of care illustrates repeatedly that the majority of informal care, especially long-term care, is provided by family rather than the wider community. Secondly, the evidence suggests that 'family care' more often than not, means care by women (Walker 1982).

On the first point, a survey by the Office of Population and Census Surveys (OPCS) in 1978 revealed that the majority of help for elderly or disabled people came from someone in the home – usually a family member. Allan in a 1987 study found that friends generally provided minimal care such as emotional support in times of crisis (Allan 1987). Allan found that care provided by friends was limited by social norms governing relationships between friends. In particular, Allan found that friendship tended to be based on *reciprocity*. Hence, friends did not like to receive more than they could give or vice versa. Friendship was also limited by the value normally placed on privacy between friends which prevented friends from providing care in terms of personal hygiene or regular meals. Likewise, Abrams *et al.* (in Snaith 1989) revealed that relationships between neighbours were governed by normality or values placed on reciprocity and privacy. Thus, neighbours occasionally helped out with simple tasks such as taking care of pets or keeping a spare key, but that regular, long-term or intimate care was not considered the proper role of neighbours.

On the second point, the General Household Survey (GHS) of 1980 revealed that 55 per cent of informal carers were women, 35 per cent of carers were male whilst in 10 per cent of cases there was disagreement about who provided most care. Likewise Abbott and Wallace in a 1990 study suggest that 75 per cent of all adults caring informally for elderly or disabled people are women (Abbott and Wallace 1990) whilst a recent survey of rural carers by the

National Federation of Women's Institutes (NFWI) found that 87 per cent of carers responding to the survey were women (NFWI 1993).

The informal provision of care has been the subject of several theoretical interpretations within the sociology of the family. The classic interpretation derives from *functionalism* in the work of such theorists as Parsons (1951) and Berger and Berger (1983). According to the functionalist interpretation of the family, women derive satisfaction and a purpose in life via the expressive roles of caring wife and mother (Wilson 1985). As a consequence of this social harmony, those receiving care get the highest quality care. The family contributes to harmony in society by being the seat of care for those in need whilst those providing care are fulfilled.

KEY TERMS

Functionalism

A theory or explanatory model in sociology. Use of a biological analogy is the simplest way to understand functionalism. Hence, just as a biologist might be concerned to understand the functioning of an organism such as a human body, the functionalist is concerned to understand the functioning of society. The functionalist studies the different parts or institutions of society to establish how these contribute to the harmonious running of the whole society.

This functionalist analysis is echoed in Conservative party political rhetoric about 'the family' (Walker 1982) but has been subject to criticism from feminists who have argued that women are trapped by a *patriarchal* society which leaves them in a subordinate position for which they are not biologically or socially predestined as the functionalists would argue. The family as an institution has been attacked by feminists as one of the most important seats of female subordination and oppression. The family has also been criticised by radical psychologists such as Laing (1971) who studied dysfunctions of the family. According to Laing such dysfunctions include tensions and hostilities which have a detrimental effect on the mental health of carers and cared for.

KEY TERMS

Patriarchy

A patriarchal system is one in which men are dominant and women are subordinate.

The impact of informal care

Ungerson (1987) suggested that it is possible to identify two broad types of carer. The first type of carer finds the experience of caring rewarding and satisfying; a certain contentment was gained. Ungerson explains this standpoint using *Freudian theory*: women (and available statistics suggest that the majority of carers are women) achieve their feminine identity and thereby satisfaction of their needs as women, through intimate and caring relationships.

KEY TERMS

Freudian theory

Freud proposed that males and females develop different gender identities according to the nature of their relationships with others. Men develop their masculine identity by establishing independence and individuality and by distancing themselves from their mothers. Women develop a feminine identity through relationships characterised by intimacy and attachment.

The second type of carer identified by Ungerson found the experience of caring depressing. These carers felt morally or practically obliged to care. Similarly the study by the National Federation of Women's Institutes (NFWI 1993) reported that four out of five carers felt that they did not have a choice about whether to take on the caring role. Ungerson finds that this perceived obligation to care translated to feelings of being trapped and of being unable to work or take part in the world outside the home. These carers felt that they had lost their identity through having to care and that their needs as people had become subordinate to the needs of someone else.

A study by Sainsbury and Grad de Alarcon (1974) suggested that informal care can affect the health of the carer. Of those families who were caring for a person with learning disabilities in the home, 60 per cent said that they had been affected mentally and 28 per cent reported being affected physically. Again, the NFWI survey provides more recent evidence. Of all carers reporting in the NFWI survey, 59 per cent reported being tired, 52 per cent were stressed, 33 per cent were emotionally exhausted and 33 per cent were suffering back trouble as a consequence of caring (NFWI 1993). The NFWI also report social impacts: 58 per cent of carers had given up their freedom, 56 per cent had given up going out, 48 per cent had given up holidays and travel whilst 15 per cent reported having given up all leisure time. These studies suggest that providing care in an informal capacity often has a sizeable impact on the life of the carer.

The impact of informal care for the person being cared for has been studied rather less but a study by Brown et al. (1972) suggested that the nature of informal care has a vital impact on the well-being of the receiver of care. It was revealed in their study that the likelihood of relapse of schizophrenic patients being discharged from hospital depended on certain factors associated with informal care provided. These factors included critical comments made by family members, expression of hostility towards the patient, expression of warmth towards the patient and level of emotional involvement with the patient. Clearly effective informal care is centrally predicated on good relationships between the carer and the person for whom the care is being provided.

CONCLUSION

Social trends in Britain today cast doubt on traditional notions of the family and community. The nuclear family is no longer widespread, nor is the traditional, caring, sharing community. Consequently, the scope for health care delivered informally by family and community is limited. The available evidence indicates that, when such care is delivered, it is delivered predominantly by women. Yet changing social roles are challenging the equity of this situation. Nevertheless government initiative continues to encourage greater provision by the informal sector and many people give and receive informal care. This care appears to have a substantial impact on the life of the giver and receiver.

EXERCISES

1 How has the nature of family and community changed over the past 100 years? Indicate possible implications of these changes for the role of the family and community in providing care.

2 Discuss evidence concerning the role that families and communities play in the provision of informal care. What are the implications of this evidence for those who provide informal care and for those who receive it?

3 Explain what is meant by the term 'ageing population' and describe demographic factors which have contributed to the existence of an ageing population in Britain in the 1990s.

4 With the use of some empirical evidence *describe* and *explain* the changing sizes and structures of families in modern Britain.

5 Assess the apparent discrepancy between the ideal of family and community care and the reality for carers.

Guided Reading

Wilson (1985) offers a clear, informed and compact introduction to the sociology of the family. The book covers sociological theories of the family and the issue of the changing family is explored. Likewise, Haralambos (1985) provides an accessible introduction to key sociological themes. The latest annual edition of *Social Trends* always provides information and figures about a multitude of relevant issues surrounding health, family and community. On the issue of caring, Ungerson (1987) explores the experience of caring from the standpoint of the carer. Similarly, the 1993 National Federation of Women's Institutes' Report makes interesting reading about the common experiences of carers.

Chapter 3

Health care and society

- Graham Moon

- Health care before 1500

- Cartesian theory

- The Development of modern medicine

- The Evolution of mental health care

- Non-medical health care

AIM

This chapter presents a brief thematic history of medical and other forms of health care. It aims to show the continuities which have led to the present biomedical health care system.

T HE PAST TWO CHAPTERS have examined health in modern Britain. The discussion has considered how present health status has evolved over time and has examined some of the factors influencing health today. It was emphasised that much of the discussion reflected a rather simplistic notion of health; it focused predominantly on disease and death. The introduction to this book represented this perspective as biomedical and not holistic. In this chapter attention turns to health care and an examination of the reasons why the health care system which dominates in modern Britain is characterised by a biomedical view of health.

The chapter is essentially a very concise and selective historical examination of British health care from approximately 1600 to the present day. In contrast to traditional medical histories the material will be presented in a way which will facilitate the understanding of developments today, rather than the detail of historical change. The chapter will also endeavour to avoid an overt reliance on dates and 'great discoveries' and the people who made them. Such material is readily available and contributes to a general impression that medical history is a matter of heroic discovery and continuous progress; the 'reality' is one of controversy, debate and, frequently, a lack of progress.

1600: competing legacies

Three competing positions on health care can be identified as existing in the late medieval period. Arguably the most powerful in a contemporary sense was a *theological* or *personalistic* perspective which saw sickness as the verdict of God upon the lifestyle of an individual. In this model health care was equated with spiritual care and a sick person could seek to become well through appropriate religious submission. Prayer, pilgrimage and the priesthood were the key elements and agents in this system.

KEY TERMS

Naturalistic health care system

A health care system dominated by a belief that ill health results from natural phenomena and can be cured or cared for by understanding those phenomena. Refers to nature and the 'natural' nature of disease.

Personalistic health care system

A health care system in which a person is both the explanation and the potential solution to a health problem. The 'person' is often a god-figure.

Alternative *naturalistic* beliefs were condemned as heresy and attempts to subvert God's will; they attracted charges of witchcraft and sorcery. Naturalistic beliefs included a *herbal tradition* and a *Graeco-Roman legacy*. Both were, to an extent, interrelated. The herbal tradition, as the name suggests, focused on the use of herbs and potions to address sickness. The knowledge necessary to deliver such health care was typically held by women and herbal care was probably the most widely practised form of health care. Graeco-Roman medicine, as developed in ancient Greece and in the Roman empire, was a naturalistic system which explained sickness from the standpoint of the balance of four 'humours': blood, black bile, yellow bile and phlegm. When one or more of the humours moved out of balance with the body, a state of sickness would result. The concept carried echoes of notions still current in Chinese and Indian medicine and, indeed, can be equated with the biomedical concept of homeostasis.

Graeco-Roman health care focused on the restoration of humouric balance; much of the herbal tradition retained vestiges of this concept but two perspectives can be drawn directly from Graeco-Roman medicine. In the *Asclepian* tradition, named after the Greek god of healing, Asclepius, the emphasis was on the use of surgery and herbs as primitive drugs. Humoural imbalances would be corrected by intervention: either by removal of the offending part or by appropriate herbal remedies. In contrast, the *Hygeian* tradition stressed lifestyle, cleanliness and rational living. Health reflected people's way of life and the conditions in which they lived; sickness could be addressed by improving these circumstances. Originally equal, the two traditions began to separate in Roman times when increasing knowledge about the internal structure of the body brought greater effectiveness to Asclepian medicine.

KEY TERMS

Asclepian tradition

An emphasis on surgery and intervention using drugs. May well involve invasion of the body; equated with cure.

Hygeian tradition: 'hygiene'

A stress on cleanliness, harmony and a sensible lifestyle; equated with care.

It is possible to trace a number of interesting contrasts in these two Graeco-Roman traditions. First, there is an embryonic separation of cure (Asclepian) from care (Hygeian). Second, there is arguably a basis to the gender division of health care: Hygeia, the Greek goddess of health, became subservient to Asclepius. In turn, Hygeian concerns became seen as less manly and less advanced. Third, in the development of the Asclepian tradition in Roman times, there is evidence for the emerging focus of medicine on the acquiring of empirical knowledge and the growing importance of seeing health as something which should be understood by knowledge of what goes on inside the body.

Cartesian theory

Graeco-Roman medical knowledge was effectively lost outside the Arab world following the fall of the Roman empire. It was rediscovered during the Renaissance period of the fifteenth and sixteenth centuries. At the time it was, of course, like herbal medicine, dangerous knowledge; it challenged the dominant role of the Church in medieval society. It was, however, increasingly shown to be effective knowledge and a good basis for addressing sickness. The critical conceptual leap – *dualism* – which enabled Graeco-Roman knowledge to be accepted and developed stemmed itself from the emerging conception of the body as a series of parts. René Descartes (1590–1650, after whom Cartesian theory is named) argued that, while the body was undoubtedly physical, it could be conceptually separated from the mind, a metaphysical and immortal element. The body and the growing knowledge of its internal architecture could safely be the realm of human physicians; the Church and religion could focus on the mind (Rose *et al.* 1984).

Two further concepts characterised the emerging medicine of the early seventeenth century. It was becoming *reductionist* and *mechanistic*. As was noted in the previous paragraph, the body was increasingly seen as a set of parts which fitted together to produce the healthy individual. Inquiry focused on identifying these parts in ever greater detail and discovering the mechanisms by which each part worked. Thus the body came to be seen as a machine driven by the heart. The sick person was a faulty machine which could be repaired by the physician or body-mechanic possessing adequate knowledge.

KEY TERMS

Reductionist
Seeing a problem or an issue as made up of a number of clearly identified parts.

Mechanistic
Explaining the origin of a problem by a machine analogy; 'the machine breaks down'.

Cartesian dualism
The separation of the mind from the body.

As a consequence of reductionism and mechanisation, health care began to focus on issues which were observable, amenable to measurement and open to accurate description. Abstract concepts like fear, feelings and attitudes began to disappear from the realm of health care; they had little place in the emerging science of the time and, to this day, some would argue that medical thought is sometimes overly detached from the human realities of sickness. It might also be argued that Cartesian theory replaced one personalistic health care system with another: one based on the scientific agency of the physician.

The emergence of modern medicine

Jewson (1976) has produced an excellent analysis recognising three major viewpoints that succeeded each other as modern medicine developed. Although Cartesian theory ultimately laid the basis for scientific medicine, it was not accepted immediately, nor was the new medicine immediately available to all. Up until the late eighteenth century the rediscovered Graeco-Roman medicine was the prerogative of a privileged few; wealthy patrons or clients might retain the services of a physician whose knowledge base was grounded in classic humoural theory. Although successful cures undoubtedly enhanced the reputation of a physician, the expertise and competence of the physician would be judged more by his (they were men) panache and social skills than his therapeutic and diagnostic success. Jewson terms this 'bedside medicine'.

Bedside medicine was based centrally on patronage. The physician might have a small number of aristocratic patients and would, effectively, be in their service and dependent on their continued patronage for an income. A consequence of this servant relationship was that bedside physicians had few opportunities to advance their skills. Diagnosis was based on the total condition of the patient and reflected only what could be seen or what the patron was willing or able to describe to the physician. The patron might even propose the treatment they wished to receive – or more often, the treatment they were prepared to tolerate. Internal examination was very rare; it would have involved a servant trespassing on the body of the patron.

By the early years of the nineteenth century, the mechanistic medical approach was beginning to be applied in medical schools.

A committed group of practitioners began to emerge and found, in the hospitals of the time, an excellent basis for extending their knowledge (Waddington 1973). Contemporary hospitals were unpleasant places; they housed people who could not afford a bedside physician to treat them at home and who were beyond the reach of herbal folk medicine. They were characterised by particularly high mortality. In France the liberalisation of autopsy legislation enabled doctors to learn about the pathology of disease by examining dead bodies; hospital doctors found themselves with an endless supply of research material which they could use to link external symptoms to internal pathology.

The emergence of what Jewson called 'hospital medicine' can be seen as the root of the dominance of the hospital in modern health care systems and the establishment of health professionals, particularly doctors, who work in hospitals as the shock troops of biomedicine. Within the hospitals, the period also saw the growth of specialism; the rate of growth of knowledge meant that it was no longer possible for a person to specialise in the whole of the body; a focus on different organs evolved with an individual only claiming expert knowledge on, for example, the kidney or the heart. The result was a transformation in medicine: the patient or client was no longer the focus of attention. Interest had been transferred to the organ and the physician was able to miss out the person. This had the effect of depersonalising health care and stressing a concern for cure at the expense of care.

The full flowering of the mechanistic and reductionist perspective is provided by Jewson's third category: 'laboratory medicine'. Reductionism now disassembled the patient/client to the component cells and tissues, not merely to organs. The sick person in the hospital bed was no longer the focus of health care, nor was the painstaking surgical investigation of his/her body. The central focus was now the pathology which could only be revealed by the laboratory test. This 'focused gaze' led to increasing specialisation among the medical profession and a growing stress on training in the scientific disciplines which provided the basis for laboratory knowledge; clinical diagnosis was increasingly structured around the requirements of the laboratory and the application of tests and technical procedures.

An important adjunct to the rise of laboratory medicine was the acceptance of the 'germ theory'. This postulated that disease resulted from the introduction of virulent micro-organisms into the body. Many of the more heroic accounts of medical history lay particular emphasis on the discoveries which underpinned this acceptance. Two further concepts were linked to the germ theory in establishing laboratory medicine as a period of seemingly remarkable success. Specific aetiology held that each disease had a single and sole cause; these causes were biomedical and related to the internal malfunctioning of the body. Their treatment involved the concept of the 'magic bullet', a treatment which would attack the cause but otherwise have no effect.

Laboratory medicine and its associated concepts has been widely seen as the zenith of the scientific approach to medicine. Its influences were rapidly absorbed in medical training and coloured the popular understanding of medicine. The progress of the epidemiological transition (see Chapter 1) at the same time has been widely seen as evidence of its success. It would be uncharitable to suggest that, at least in part, this was not the case although, as McKeown (1979) has argued and Chapter 1 has demonstrated, the work of the nineteenth-century sanitary reformers was probably of greater importance to the vast majority of people through its creation of cleaner living conditions and reduced overcrowding. see p. 23 However, the purely scientific model undoubtedly contributed to some neglect of the social and spiritual aspects of people care. It also, despite the contemporary activity of sanitary reformers, engendered a suggestion that cure, treatment and repair were all-important and that internal medical intervention was somehow better than social, environmental and psychological care.

Medicine today

Today the laboratory medicine approach has been modified. It is recognised that diseases generally have many causes and that care is at least the equal of cure. Although biomedical ideas continue to dominate modern notions of health care, social and psychological approaches are increasingly recognised. Today's health care system is multi-national, industrial and complex (Berliner 1985). A major role is played by the companies which manufacture drugs and medical technology. These operate on a multi-national scale, selling their wares across the globe and structuring the way in which medicine develops. The industrial epithet stems from the way in which cures and treatment protocols are increasingly standardised, technology has come to dominate many specialties, and patients/ clients are increasingly processed in a semi-industrial way; contemporary terminology which refers to workload and throughput substantiates this point. Complexity is reflected in the increasing fragmentation of the health care process. The ever-growing number of specialties are a confirmation of this point.

The emergence of the medico-industrial complex has had a number of consequences. First, it has brought about a differential ranking of specialisms. Those specialisms which employ the full panoply of technical and scientific approaches have gained more acclaim than those which do not; thus surgery is ranked above the care of elderly people. Second, the pre-eminence of the hospital has been unchallenged. Only very recently has home care re-emerged onto the health care agenda as the high cost of hospital care and its limitations have become apparent. Third, health care has expanded. Social problems have been *medicalised*; reconstructed as medical problems with medical intervention represented as a solution to these problems. Most obviously this last point is evident in the increasing expectations regarding medical care as a treatment for mental health problems, such as depression, which may stem more from social isolation than any fundamental bio-medical base (Conrad and Schneider 1980).

Beyond acute care

So far this brief history of health care has focused heavily on acute medicine. Little has been said about care for people with mental health problems or people with learning difficulties. The history of care for both these groups is somewhat different from the evolution of general medical care, although some parallels can be drawn (Busfield 1986). In both cases, the differences reveal much about the limits of medicine and also the difficulty of making a division between health and social care.

Notwithstanding the recent existence of large hospitals for both people with mental health problems and people with learning difficulties, the traditional mode of care for both groups was the family. Families would have been expected to provide care for their less fortunate members. Some church care might have been available for those unable to afford to care. Family care would have been unlikely to be medicalised and would generally have simply taken the form of protection, clothing, feeding and comfort. Within the community as a whole, there would have been a mixture of tolerance, providing 'the problem' was managed within the family, and exclusion of the more frightening aspects of mental ill health.

The historical process which led to the Cartesian revolution had consequences in the world of mental health care and the care of people with learning difficulties. Once the paternalistic notion of God's punishment had been opened to challenge, it was perhaps inevitable that a movement would develop designed to meet that challenge. In the mental health and learning difficulties fields that movement owed considerable debts to the Hygeian tradition; it also, perhaps more importantly, reflected a growing societal move to exclude people who were 'different' from the main body of society (see Chapters 5 and 8 for a discussion of the notion of stigma). The result was the growth of the asylum movement.

Prior to the growth of asylums, family care had been increasingly replaced by institutional care. As people with mental health problems and people with learning difficulties did not, by and large, earn incomes, they were dependent on the primitive social support systems of the times. These comprised the workhouses, institutions which could house anyone who was temporarily or permanently without paid work – the poor, the mad, the criminal. The Hygeian aspect to the growth of the asylums was that they were intended to provide improving therapeutic environments, asylums, where people might come to terms with and perhaps recover from their problem. At the same time, the asylums also served the purpose of excluding people; they were typically located on the outskirts of towns or in rural settings behind high walls.

Asylums today have a generally dreadful reputation. Yet they were founded with the best of intentions. These good intentions were progressively undone through the nineteenth and the first half of the twentieth centuries. They became overcrowded and the therapeutic conditions, which had originally included space for each resident, were removed. The treatment regimes became progressively less enlightened and more custodial. There were also cross-linkages with the emergence of laboratory medicine; certainly mental health care became heavily dependent on drug and electro-mechanical therapies. By the mid-twentieth century, commentators such as Goffman (1991), were able to document, at length, the effective failure of the asylum system to function in a therapeutic way. Much of this criticism focused on the degrading and inhumane treatment of clients. The original small private asylums had been overtaken by large public asylums funded by towns as little more than warehouses for their less fortunate citizens.

At the same time as the failings of the asylums were being documented, other factors were also emerging. First, the majority of the large public asylums had been built in the mid- to late nineteenth century. By the mid-twentieth century their fabric was decaying and they were falling down. The repair bill to maintain them was growing rapidly. Second, the cost of nursing and treating the population of people in the asylums was growing. Third, the progress of laboratory medicine and the emergence of the medico-industrial complex had ensured that drug treatments had developed for some mental health problems. These drug therapies meant that a person with a mental health problem no longer had to live permanently in a health care setting. Taken together, these factors – a combination of cost-containment, drug development and therapeutic enlightenment – enabled the emergence of community care and a retreat from the asylum-based mode of residential care.

Today community care is the norm in both mental health and learning difficulties services. It is perceived as the best and most effective way of providing care and the emphasis is on social and caring aspects rather than on the medicalisation of these areas. Yet residential care has neither been completely abandoned nor wholly discredited. It is recognised that there is a clear group of clients for whom community care is simply impossible. For some their needs are too extensive; others have lived for so long in residential care that discharge would be inhumane. A not insignificant private residential care sector has also continued to exist. There is also a recognition that, contrary to some initial misconceptions, community care has not proved to be a cheap option. It has required and continues to require considerable investment in order to work effectively.

see pp. 170–72

Beyond the doctors

So far this chapter has talked generally of health care. Where specific health professionals have been discussed, they have generally been doctors. Hopefully, a careful reading of the preceding sections will have revealed *why* the medical profession has become central to discussions of health care: its dominance can be traced right back to the submission of the Hygeian to the Asclepian tradition. Its progress to dominance is inextricably linked to the process of reductionism and mechanisation and to the establishment of medicine as 'scientific'. In this final section to the present chapter the discussion is extended to consider health care professions other than medicine.

In considering health care professions other than medicine we must confront the gender division evident in health care work. Although the situation is changing and there have always been some anomalies, it has generally been the case that doctors have been men and members of other health care professions have been women. This too can be traced to the Hygeian–Asclepian separation. Men chose the public, intellectual, scientific and, after the advances of hospital and laboratory medicine, the financially lucrative world of doctoring. Women were limited by social role to the private domestic role of caring and hygiene maintenance. Although this role may have been limiting in one sense, the shortcomings, poor record and lack of availability of medicine meant that, for most people women were, nevertheless, the dominant carers. As Barbara Ehrenreich and Deirdre English have argued:

> Women have always been healers. They were the unlicensed doctors and anatomists of western history. They were the abortionists, doctors and counsellors. They were the pharmacists, cultivating healing herbs and exchanging the secrets of their uses. They were the midwives travelling from home to home and village to village.
>
> (Ehrenreich and English 1976)

An alternative Hygeian health care tradition was therefore maintained, practised by women. The history of the health care professions other than medicine is largely, though not exclusively, a history of the accommodation of this tradition with scientific medicine while, at the same time, being a history of gender relations in which a male-dominated profession has identified acceptable boundaries to women's activities.

Nursing provides an excellent example of these processes at work (Dingwall *et al.* 1988). As hospital medicine developed into laboratory medicine, the lack of educational opportunities for women effectively excluded them from the medical profession. Nor did contemporary society expect women to enter professions such as medicine. Those women who were involved in health care were involved as nurses who were little more than comforters and helpers. To this role they brought the traditional skills as carers alluded to above. At least until the middle of the nineteenth century they also brought these skills from largely working-class environments where standards of cleanliness and hygiene were often far below those expected by the middle-class scientifically trained doctors. Consequently the reputation of nurses was generally poor.

The Nightingale reforms changed this situation. They re-created nursing as a suitable profession for middle-class single women. The new nurses of the time were recruited predominantly in elite hospitals where they practised as helpers to doctors of whom they were the social, if not educational, equal. While the standard of nursing had undoubtedly been raised, nineteenth-century standards of gender equality still prevailed. Indeed it is probably fair to say that the Nightingale reforms, through their success and their longlasting impact, were instrumental in maintaining the nursing elements of health care in a subordinate position to the medical aspects for at least a century.

Nursing is, of course, not a single homogeneous group. While the Nightingale reforms linked general nursing firmly into the frame of laboratory medicine, those nurses working outside the elite hospitals in the Poor Law institutions and asylums catering for people with mental health problems and people with learning difficulties continued to be recruited from lower-status groups and to work in a correspondingly lower status and more custodial environment. The most striking difference between these nurses and the Nightingale elite were that they tended to be male, reflecting the emphasis on physical skills of restraint.

The move to community care identified in the previous section changed this situation. Not only did it open up the asylums to scrutiny which had inevitable consequences for the model of care, it also exposed the practices of staff to those of other agencies responsible for the welfare of the client population. Thus the caring aspect of nursing in the areas of mental health and learning difficulties developed rapidly and cross-fertilisation with the practices of social care agencies developed apace. Perhaps not unexpectedly women began to enter these two areas of nursing practice in greater numbers.

CONCLUSION

This chapter has endeavoured to present a thematic social history of health care. A great deal of material and a vast sweep of time have been covered in a very small space. Inevitably the chapter has been general and broad in its assertions and suggestions, while stressing the importance of the social context of historical development. The general tenor of the chapter has been critical. Medicine has been portrayed as a process which has evolved towards a cure-centred perspective from which people have been excluded. Question marks have been placed over its relations with women. However, there are, of course, immense achievements in medical history. Few people today would wish to live in a world without anaesthesia, vaccinations and modern drugs, yet there are times when the caring element of modern health care seems to be secondary.

EXERCISES

1 Although this chapter has argued that medical history should not be seen as a series of great events, it usually is! Make yourself a list of major medical discoveries noting the date, discoverer and implications of each discovery.

2 What have been the consequences of laboratory medicine for modern health care?

3 Discuss the relationship between the medical profession and another health care profession of your choice. Identify the good and bad aspects of the relationship and assess their consequences.

Guided Reading

Open University (1985a) is an excellent concise history of the material covered in this chapter. A more focused account of the historical development of nursing is provided by Dingwall *et al.* (1988).

Chapter 4

Criticisms of biomedicine

- Chloe Gerhardt

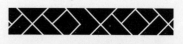

- **Critiques of biomedicine**

  - environmental

  - public health

  - feminist

  - Marxist

  - philosophical

Six critics of biomedicine are looked at, chosen because their views have presented challenging arguments concerning biomedical provision. An examination of their views introduces a variety of different perspectives found within the social sciences on the relationship between medicine and health.

HISTORICALLY THERE HAS BEEN A DICHOTOMY between the ideas of cure and care when examining concepts of health. This has been termed 'the never-ending oscillation between two different points of view in medicine' (Dubos 1960). These different points of view have concerned the necessity to achieve balance between the body, the mind and the environment and, against this, the determination to intervene directly in the process of disease. As the previous chapter argued, the recent history of health care has led to solutions to health problems being sought in the first instance through a biomedical interventionist approach.

There has been increasing criticism from the 1960s onwards, both from those working within the health system and from those outside it, that this pre-eminent position attained by biomedicine requires close and critical examination. This chapter examines these criticisms of biomedicine through an analysis of the key published works of a selection of important critics. The books which have been selected provide arguments which focus on Britain, Europe, America, and the developing world, showing how biomedical services may sometimes fail to meet health needs, and encourage unsuitable or even damaging approaches to health. Consideration of these alternatives to the standard view about the medical model provides a valuable critical perspective on the current health care.

René Dubos

To ward off disease or recover health, men as a rule find it easier to depend on healers than to attempt the more difficult task of living wisely.

(Dubos, quoted in Black *et al.* 1987)

The first of the critics to be examined in this chapter is René Dubos, an American microbiologist (Dubos 1960). To him the

see p. 57

doctrine of specific aetiology is only a partial explanation of the cause of disease because it cannot explain the conditions under which this aetiology may be found. Thus, while a specific micro-organism may well 'cause' a disease, Dubos would be interested in the conditions under which the micro-organism would flourish.

Dubos argued that, throughout history, there have been differing meanings given to health. Consequently, ideas about how to maintain or create health have changed, swinging between practices which favour preventive 'healthy living' approaches, and those emphasising curative, disease-focused measures. To decide that the biomedical approach is suitable in all circumstances, for all people, is unwise, since the world is constantly changing, and living things, according to Dubos, 'can survive and function effectively only if they adapt themselves to the peculiarities of each individual situation' (Dubos, quoted in Black *et al.* 1987). New health threats are constantly created, so medicine must adapt and find new and socially responsive ways of tackling suffering and disease.

Holistic approaches to health find resonance with such criticism, because they are concerned with finding ways of dealing with sickness and disease through gaining greater understanding of individuals, the contexts in which they live, their social and mental states, and their own beliefs. Remedies can then be tailored to this information, for this person, rather than tied to the specific aetiology and applied to all. Environmentalists similarly have given Dubos credit for stressing that human beings adapt to their environments best when changing health needs are incorporated into medical care.

Dubos is not calling for radical changes, because he believes that medicine should not be identified with political action, although he does implicate the way that society is organised in the production of illness (Jones and Moon 1987: 24). The strength of his criticisms is based on his lengthy historical analysis of changing approaches to health and disease He uses this to provide evidence of the inability of biomedicine to cope with present-day illness and disease. It is adaptability and a knowledge of the relationship between people and their environments which he believes are required rather than what he sees as the rigidity of biomedicine.

Archie Cochrane

> I believe that cure is rare while the need for care is wide-
> spread, and that the pursuit of cure at all costs may restrict
> the supply of care.
>
> (Cochrane 1972: 7)

Cochrane's experience as a doctor, starting his career in the economic
depression of the 1930s, made him convinced that universal provision through the National Health Service was of enormous potential benefit to health, but that much of medicine's reputation rested
on untested assumptions (Cochrane 1972). Having been a senior
medical officer in a prisoner of war camp with little medical provision yet few deaths among the often sick inmates, he also retained
a conviction that medicine must acknowledge and utilise the importance of the recuperative power of the human body.

Cochrane's central contribution to the critique of biomedicine
centred around his concern about untested assumptions. He
deplored the absence of cost/benefit considerations which would
enable analysis of the 'effectiveness' and 'efficiency' of medical care.
He argued for clinical randomised control trials (RCTs) as a
rigorous scientific means of evaluating medical procedures, some
of which, he alleged, had little proven value. He also argued that
a proper examination of effectiveness and efficiency should take
account of social inequalities.

KEY TERMS

Randomised control trials (RCTs)

Enable the 'testing of a hypothesis that a certain treatment
alters the natural history of a disease for the better' (Cochrane
1972:20). They involve the random allocation of people to one
of two groups: one which receives a treatment and one which
does not. Statistically significant differences between the two
groups indicate that claims for the effectiveness of the treatment are not simply the result of chance.

Cochrane does not suggest that there is anything seriously wrong with the traditional lines of health service and medical research. The power of his criticisms comes from the implication inherent in his claim that much of what was done in the name of medicine was untested, unsupportable, inequitable, and consequently determined by the interests of the medical profession, rather than the needs of the patients. In writing his critique Cochrane was making a plea for the British National Health Service to improve its effectiveness and efficiency. His criticisms related not just to standards of care, but to the potential financial wastage. He was well ahead of his time in raising such issues, many of which are now central for reformers of health care, although he was primarily concerned with NHS's ability to identify and meet the needs of patients rather than with reducing costs.

Thomas McKeown

Contrary to what is generally believed, the most fundamental issue confronting medical science is not the solution of one or more of the unsolved biomedical problems: it is evaluation of two approaches to the control of disease, one through understanding of mechanisms and the other through a knowledge of origins.

(McKeown 1979:166)

McKeown wrote as a medical doctor and demographer. He took a historical look at medical practice, and argued that there should be a recognition of the limited impact of medical procedures on the overall health of the population. Thus, as argued in Chapter 1, the decline in infectious diseases and the growth of the population were, for McKeown, only partially due to medical progress. see p. 25 Furthermore, he suggested that the possibly exaggerated role of medicine had led to significant over-investment in medical approaches to health care. McKeown claimed that it was social changes which made the major health impact on infectious diseases. In particular, he cited improvements in nutritional status, and better living conditions as the key factors involved in limiting the impact of infectious disease. In the case of chronic and intractable health conditions, he argued for the importance of individual lifestyle decisions; he suggested that personal behaviour is now becoming a predominant determinant of health.

Lifestyle

In a health studies context lifestyle generally refers to health-related behaviours. A standard analysis sees four such behaviours: eating, drinking, smoking, and exercise. To these are sometimes added health care utilisation behaviour, sexuality and sexual behaviour, and substance misuse. Each 'lifestyle' is linked to particular health problems.

McKeown's conclusions have policy implications for public health, for benefit levels, and for health-promotion strategies. Medicine, to be of greatest value, must consequently concern itself with investigating the origins and mechanisms of disease. With nearly all the non-fatal diseases, where there are no wholly effective treatments, medicine should concentrate on relieving discomfort, and not make greater claims. If medicine is to be effective, McKeown argues, it should be concerned with prevention as well as treatment, with care as well as cure, and with the context of sickness as well as intervention: he states that the institution of medicine should be 'concerned with all the influences on health' (McKeown 1979: ix). This conclusion is exemplified particularly clearly by reference to one of McKeown's own key examples: the decline in respiratory tuberculosis. This disease, despite being a medical success story, is now being diagnosed as on the increase again among those whose social conditions leave them vulnerable.

Ann Oakley

It is from the 'scientific' representations of women as maternity cases that the character of mothers is deduced. 'Science'

71

has hidden curricula of moral evaluations that masquerade as fact.

(Oakley 1980: 5)

The feminist movement has provided many studies which analyse the way in which the largely male-dominated medical profession has been able to manipulate and define women's roles and problems. An example of such a contribution, from a sociological perspective, is Ann Oakley's book *Women Confined*, in which she investigates the experience of childbirth (Oakley 1980). In her book she is critical not just of the medical profession but of sociological investigations of reproduction which omit the actual experience of women themselves, concentrating rather on statistical analysis, and 'the cultural idealization of femininity and maternity' (Oakley 1980: 90).

Oakley examines childbirth through a series of extended interviews carried out with women expecting their first babies. She argues for childbirth to be seen as a life event similar to other changes in life, even though it carries physical, emotional, psychological and social implications, particularly when it is the first childbirth. Reproduction has profound effects on the lives of women. It is 'an experience of control by medical professionals, of birth by technology and surgery, with the mother as passive subject rather than active agent' (Oakley 1980: 257). What should be life events can frequently result in undermining self-esteem and depression. Women, she argues, should be able to look at childbirth as a genuine achievement, which is able to 'endow a lasting legacy of self-respect and belief in self-determination' (Oakley 1980: 300).

Oakley's study used the technique of 'phenomenology' and places the accounts she generated into a feminist framework which valued the perspectives of women rather than those of the often male medical establishment. She provides both a powerful critique of medical practice as applied to pregnant women, and a useful outline of a sociological method of investigation which gives priority to the views of women themselves. Consumerism within the National Health Service is now attempting to find ways in which such views can be responded to within maternity services. Midwives themselves are fighting for extending their right to make decisions about pregnancy and childbirth with the women concerned, rather than these being dominated and dictated by the medical profession.

Phenomenology

An approach to research and understanding which examines everyday accounts and understandings by people involved in the subject of study.

Vincente Navarro

The underdevelopment of health ... is not due to prevalent lifestyles – as behavioural theorists indicate – but rather to the dramatic maldistribution of economic and political power in our society.

(Navarro 1976: xi)

From a Marxist perspective, any critique of biomedicine has to be placed within the broader context of the role of the capitalist state within which it is practised. The intention is to set 'the tree' (the health sector), within the setting of 'the forest' (the economic and political structure) (Navarro 1976: 165). And as the influences of capitalism are international, many Marxists place their criticisms within the international setting.

Marxist perspectives

There are many different forms of Marxism; all purport to follow the basic thinking of Karl Marx, a nineteenth-century economic philosopher. The essential element of Marxism is the belief that many issues can be analysed in terms of the relation between capital (basically wealth and money) and labour (the work needed to produce capital). The capitalist system is an example of a social and political system which operates to benefit those who own the firms and institutions in which labour is done. In a health context, such a system needs a healthy workforce.

The American Marxist Vincente Navarro's book *Medicine Under Capitalism* (Navarro 1976) is concerned with the way in which there is a close relationship between the nature of the state and health. Similar, though more measured, claims are made by Lesley Doyal (1979) in a British context. The nature of the perspective can most clearly be seen in morbidity and mortality statistics when analysed by class and country. The economic structure of a country determines and maintains a particular class structure: 'the different degrees of ownership, control and influence that these classes have on the means of production, reproduction, and legitimization ... explain the composition, nature and functions of the health sectors' (Navarro 1976: xii). Consequently, those countries where the economies are dominated and exploited by capitalism, have health systems which reflect the needs of capital. Arguments about the most appropriate model of health care, or appropriate professional roles are misplaced: 'more important than the shape of the final product is the issue of who dominates the process' (Navarro 1976: 165).

Following this analysis, ill health under capitalism results from the impact of measures designed to enhance the profitability of capital: from shiftwork, overtime, dangerous chemicals, industrial injuries, stress, or a damaged and polluted environment. Such health-damaging factors pose the greatest threat to those in the lower social classes, the poor, and those in developing countries, because their lives are more vulnerable to the direct and cumulative effects of such capitalist processes through their close relationship to production. Biomedicine consequently has an important role to play within capitalism, as it holds responsibility for providing health services for the workers of capitalism: it helps them to maintain, or to regain their health and this enables them to play their productive roles effectively.

The Marxist analysis provides a 'macro' view: it links social, political, economic data across time and across countries, to expose the dynamics of social inequalities that can then be tackled through class and community action. In looking at medicine, the analysis is concerned with the relationship between the needs of capital and the form that medicine takes in supporting it by making workers fit to work and curing the results of work-induced sickness. Only through challenging the nature of production, that is where the profit motive is dominant, will significant changes be made in society, and in the way that biomedicine is organised and applied.

A Marxist alternative would offer a different relationship between the state and professional groups such as the medical profession. Medicine would serve social rather than class interests and its effectiveness would be determined through democratic and socialist processes, rather than being determined by the needs of capital and powerful professional groups serving these interests. Moreover, the Marxist critique makes it clear that there will be little impact on health derived from reorganising biomedical health care if the domination of capitalism is not challenged first.

Ivan Illich

Iatrogenic medicine reinforces a morbid society in which social control of the population by the medical system turns into a principal economic activity.

(Illich 1976: 51)

The criticisms that Illich presents in his book *Limits to Medicine* (Illich 1976) are substantially different from those of other critics presented in this chapter. This is because his concern is not to outline ways in which western medicine can be best utilised or expropriated so that its benefits are universal, social, equitable, effective, or efficient. His purpose is to stress the damage that western biomedicine itself is doing to society as a whole. He writes as a philosopher and theologian. The medical establishment, Illich argues, has become a major threat to health, on the scale of an epidemic. The result is what he calls 'iatrogenesis'. A definition of iatrogenesis as applied to clinical practice would be when pain, sickness and death result from medical care, but he extends this definition so that it encompasses the wider implications of relying on medical solutions to what are, in most cases, social and spiritual problems.

Illich cites a recurring theme in 'holistic' health: the need for spiritual and personal dimensions in coping with illness and disease.

Suffering, healing, and dying, which are essentially intransitive activities that culture taught each man, are now claimed by technology as new areas of policy-making and are treated

KEY TERMS

Types of iatrogenesis

Clinical – 'comprises all clinical conditions for which remedies, physicians, or hospitals are the pathogens, or "sickening" agents' (Illich 1976: 36). This includes 'the undesirable side-effects of approved, mistaken, callous, or contra-indicated technical contacts with the medical system' (Illich 1976: 41).

Social – when health policies reinforce an industrial organisation that generates ill health: medical practice sponsors sickness 'by reinforcing a morbid society that encourages people to become consumers of curative, preventive, industrial and environmental medicine' (Illich 1976: 42). By doing this, diagnosis becomes a way in which political concerns with the stresses brought about by economic and industrial growth are turned into demands for more therapies.

Cultural – through emphasising technological solutions and relief from symptoms, the social environment within which people lead their lives is deprived of conditions that give individuals, families, and neighbourhoods a means of understanding and coping with their circumstances and feelings.

as malfunctions from which populations ought to be institutionally relieved.

(Illich 1976:138)

He is concerned not with capitalism, but with the destructive processes of industrialisation. He criticises the role professionals play in undermining individual autonomy, and calls for a recognition of the value to society of the interpretations of the pain and suffering which accompany illness and death. Iatrogenesis as Illich has developed the term, provides us with a critique for examining biomedicine at all levels of social and spiritual life – its damaging effects, its palliatives, its spiritual detachment, its political non-involvement. His concerns have been taken up in many other studies which examine the abuses and false claims of biomedicine.

CONCLUSION

While the writers chosen here can be linked by the powerful arguments that they present in their criticisms of biomedicine, their opinions come from divergent positions, use different levels of analysis, and consequently have different implications. These encompass the need for more rigour in scientific method, the importance of public health, the politics of class and community struggle, the impoverishment of spiritual values, and the need to listen to personal accounts, in particular, the voices of women. They present illustrations of a range of differing social science perspectives and theories and make suggestions which cast doubt on heroic accounts of biomedicine and its claims for scientific value-freedom. At the nub of their critiques is a common recognition that care and healing is seldom accomplished through biomedicine alone.

EXERCISES

1 Complete short, paragraph-length summaries of the views of the critics of biomedicine considered in this chapter.

2 To what extent is it possible to distinguish between the critiques of biomedicine made by doctors and the critiques made from outside the medical profession?

3 What are the implications of the critiques of biomedicine for the practice of health care in Britain today?

4 Use a local academic library to examine reviews of the works of McKeown, Dubos, Cochrane, Navarro, Doyal, Illich and Oakley.

Guided Reading

Both Jones and Moon (1987) and Morgan *et al.* (1985) provide brief summaries of the critiques and critics outlined in this chapter. There is however, no substitute for a reading of the critics' key works in the original. Some of these are reproduced in Black *et al.* 1987) and McKeown (1979) and Doyal (1979) are both highly readable.

Social dimensions of sickness and disability

- Rosemary Gillespie
- Chloe Gerhardt

Chapter 5

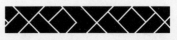

- **Models of health**

  - the medical model

  - the social model

- **Social responses to sickness**

  - the sick role

  - deviance

This chapter outlines some of the ways in which the social sciences, and sociology in particular, have sought to examine health, illness and disability. The chapter describes and contrasts the medical and social models of health, and examines sociological theories which attempt to provide a framework within which to interpret the social nature of responses to illness and disease.

I T WILL BE CLEAR from the brief look at critics of biomedicine in Chapter 4 that it is possible to draw from different disciplines and perspectives in analysing the role that medicine plays
in society. In this, the concluding chapter to the first part of this
book, the substance of these criticisms is aggregated to form the
basis of an alternative social model of health which can be set
alongside the more usual medical model of health. The chapter
then assesses the utility of the social model in promoting an understanding of sickness as a social state.

Medical and social models

The term 'biomedicine' has been used extensively in the previous
chapters. Together with its synonym, the medical model, it can be
used to identify a natural science-based medical theory and practice which focuses upon the internal workings of the body. Biomedicine is the dominant paradigm in modern western health care.
However, biomedical assumptions are now being questioned by
alternative social models of ill health which take up the critiques
and shortcomings identified in the previous chapters.

KEY TERMS

Dominant paradigm

A way of understanding and interpreting a problem which is
taken for granted and accepted by society to the virtual exclusion of other approaches. In the sense of this present text, the
term therefore refers not just to acceptance by those within
the profession of medicine, but also by society as a whole.

The two models of health are analytical tools: they show characteristics which can be used to describe the major features of two ways of identifying, interpreting and dealing with health problems. They can be deliberately posed as 'opposites', to highlight these distinctions. In reality, however, health care practice recognises the need to give consideration to social factors and is increasingly concerned with lifestyles and personal health management. Moreover, sociologists increasingly recognise the complex relationship between the biological and social. Nevertheless, it would still be true to say that there is a substantial gulf between these two ways of perceiving reality.

The scientific method is seen as central to biomedicine. Thus biomedicine works by testing theories until they can be accepted as 'facts'. Established medical 'facts' are based, not upon conjecture or supposition, but upon specific, universally accepted, rigorous procedures, which focus on the internal workings of the body, including mental processes. It is these 'facts' that provide the basis for medical practice. The social model disputes the neutrality, applicability and universality of such a world-view. It is not, however, suggested that a social model will replace the scientific one. Rather, the sociology of health and illness stresses the need to acknowledge that scientific and medical 'facts' themselves are a particular way of perceiving illness and disease. Such 'facts' deny people's own interpretations of the world and avoid any in-depth consideration of root social causes. They also deny the extent to which historical, social and cultural factors shape perceptions of reality. The scientific method itself comes in for criticism, as the case is made that it is, arguably, the professional monopoly of doctors guarding and defining what is considered 'legitimate medical knowledge', which has provided medicine with its domination over other ways of looking at illness.

The social model of health sets out a perspective, which attempts to find the root causes of disease outside the body: the social production of ill health and disease. This perspective seeks to identify those factors which will undermine or destroy the health of the individual, and which can be found in social life. The social model is based firmly on a belief that, behind the surface manifestations of disease, lie 'real' causes relating to the way in which society is organised and structured. Such causes reflect particular theoretical positions. Thus, a feminist analysis might stress such notions as patriarchy or oppression.

Medical model

- A state of health is a biological fact:
  - it is immutable, real, independent.
- Ill health is caused by biological calamities:
  - 'entrants' to the body (e.g. viruses, germs);
  - 'internal faults' (e.g. genes);
  - trauma.
- Causes are identified by:
  - signs and symptoms;
  - the process of 'diagnosis';
  - establishing deviation from medically established 'normality'.
- Medical knowledge is exclusionary:
  - it is the job of the expert or specialist;
  - facts are accumulated and built upon;
  - alternative perspectives are invalid and inferior.
- Biomedicine is reductionist and disease-oriented, concerned with pathology.

Social model

- A state of health is socially constructed:
  - it is varied, uncertain, diverse.
- Ill health is caused by social factors:
  - behind the biology lies society;
  - root causes are social causes.
- Causes are identified through:
  - beliefs, which are varying, subjective, society- and community-based;
  - interpretation, built up through custom and social constraint.
- Knowledge is not exclusionary:
  - it has a historical, cultural and social context;
  - it is shaped by involved people.
- The social model is holistic and concerned with context.

Biomedical certainty is based on an assumption that people in all their individual, spiritual and social complexity, can be 'reconstructed' or understood more profoundly through the accumulating facts about different parts of their bodies. 'Reductionism' of see p. 54 this form is problematic. It is questionable whether it is possible to comprehend the everyday dynamics of ill health when people are perceived simply as the sum or consequence of their parts. Sociological inquiry questions the adequacy of seeing health as merely the gathering of facts.

Central to the social model is a recognition of the close relationships between medical practice, the power invested in the medical profession and the particular manner in which illness and disease are defined. In biomedicine, this has traditionally been centred on finding cures rather than preventing ill health, and hospital rather than community-based approaches to care. Definitions and categories of disease and of deviance cannot, however, be seen as immutable facts once historical and cultural dimensions are considered. They are struggled over, change and represent different things to different people. Health strategies and policies must take this into account.

Making sense of health

Wendy Stainton Rogers (1991) is one of a number of writers who have explored the way in which people themselves make sense of the world when coping with their own health problems. She draws from anthropology, sociology and psychology in her research and demonstrates that people select their explanations of health and illness from a number of existing complementary explanations or accounts depending on the particular circumstances or condition, and their beliefs. These explanations include both the biomedical and the social and have a value to the individual which cannot be judged from the point of view of rationality, scientific soundness or adequacy. It is not 'authenticity' which is being sought, but personal satisfaction and comprehension. This has important implications for biomedicine – not because biomedicine is ineffective – but as a consequence of: 'the assumption that biomedicine is the *only* valid medical system, that it has some natural superiority, or that it is universally benign, morally neutral and merely "mirrors reality" without distortion' (Stainton Rogers 1991: 21).

For the remainder of this chapter attention will turn to the examination of two important sociological constructs which demonstrate the centrality of social factors to understanding the experience of health and ill health.

The sick role

Important to the linking of the analysis of social systems with the illness experiences of the individual is the concept of the *sick role*, which was first conceptualised by Parsons (1951). Parsons' sick role provides a counter to the medical model, showing that illness should not be considered as merely an event which happens naturally, which is unmotivated and therefore excluded from the sociological analysis of deviation from an expected role (Stainton Rogers 1991: 27). The sick role shows how social definitions of sickness reflect the larger cultural values of a society. Viewed from a functionalist perspective, sickness provides an example of behaviour which can be either encouraged or discouraged; punished or rewarded.

see p. 44

KEY TERMS

The sick role

The concept of the sick role is a now somewhat dated but still useful legacy of functionalist sociology. It focuses on the social role of being sick. It distinguishes:

Rights: to be exempt from normal obligations such as going to work; to receive help in order to recover.

Duties: to want to recover; to acquiesce to prescribed treatment regimes.

Within biomedicine, it is traditionally doctors who are given the licence to label patients as sick. This is done on the basis of the presenting symptoms. The doctor therefore acts as 'gatekeeper', and consequently controls access to the sick role. In this role there are clear notions of 'rights' and 'duties'. Rights arise out of the diagnosed sickness label, and duties arise from adopting the correct role in response. The rights reflect the fact that sickness is not a deliberate condition and the belief that biomedicine is the most appropriate treatment for ill health. The duties carry with them the notion that there is such a thing as 'normal functioning' – a state of being well – which should be aspired to by everyone. The duties also indicate a belief that people should relax into the sick role and submit to whatever help is given.

Essentially the sick role sees sickness as 'social deviance', rather than a scientifically diagnosed biological state. Through such a theory, expected social roles become visible, such as appropriate behaviour in doctor/patient encounters; those who can sanction or condemn resulting deviations can be identified. Through adopting the sick role when it has not been granted, prolonging it or refusing to accept advice, a member of society may be labelled as weak, a malingerer or a difficult patient. The theory can therefore be applied to medical encounters in powerful ways, and used to examine the role that the medical profession plays in defining such deviation.

Parsons' depiction of the sick role has been subjected to considerable criticism. It can, to give one of the major criticisms, be seen to have all the shortcomings that a functionalist model gives rise to because of its assumption that society is some kind of coherent social whole, protecting weaker members, held together by the checks and balances of social norms. A resulting weakness is in dealing with the inequalities of power which can be found in sick-role encounters. The functionalist view assumes that social norms are primarily determined by their ability to maintain the shape and stability of social relationships and institutions. This approach is criticised by those arguing that inequalities and disagreements and conflict are a permanent feature of society. The power that biomedicine has, for example, in effectively controlling entry to the sick role, can profoundly influence and control subsequent medical and social relationships. Furthermore the dominance of biomedicine maintains this power.

Another criticism is that the sick role cannot adequately deal with social roles which are not easy to define, such as chronic illness or mental ill health. It is more applicable to acute episodes of illness, where being in a position to re-establish a 'normal role' is expected or desired. In chronic-illness encounters, there is far more ambiguity as to when either the doctor, the patient or perhaps the employer or carer are in a position to accept the adoption of the sick role. Pregnancy also provides an example of problems which arise in trying to apply the concept of the sick role to all medical encounters. While medicalisation has resulted in the extensive involvement of the medical profession during pregnancy and the birth, there is often confusion and conflict in the social role expected of women during this period:

> Although pregnancy involves a disturbance of a biological state, and at some point a disruption of role obligations, it calls forth a set of responses, both from the woman herself and her significant others, which are in many ways different from those elicited with the onset of illness.
>
> (Morgan *et al.* 1985: 49)

The social creation of stigma

Health professionals work closely with individuals and their families, affected by a wide range of health challenges. Many illnesses, diseases and handicaps attract social reactions that evoke negative attitudes. It is important for health professionals to have an understanding of the social processes involved in the acquisition of such negative societal reaction or *stigma*. For example, health professionals, especially doctors, exercise a great deal of power when diagnosing 'socially unacceptable' diseases such as epilepsy, sexually transmitted diseases or HIV and AIDS. These diagnoses and society's reactions to them can affect a person's life and social circumstances, and have important implications for the ways in which people manage and challenge stigmatising identities ranging from illnesses and diseases to disablements and disfigurements (Williams 1987; Scambler 1989).

The term stigma comes from the Greek, referring to signs cut or burnt into the body, which exposed the bearer as a slave, a criminal or a traitor or other social outcast, who was ritually polluted and to be avoided (Goffman 1963: 11). More recently the meaning refers to a trait or condition that symbolically marks the bearer as 'culturally unacceptable' or inferior (Williams 1987: 136).

KEY TERMS

Stigma

May be defined as a negative social reaction. It also reflects social devaluation and negative labelling of individuals. Much of the sociological literature on stigma is derived from the work of Erving Goffman, who described stigma in terms of spoiled identity (Goffman 1963). Goffman's work is derived from the micro-sociological perspective, symbolic interactionism, which focuses on the face-to-face interaction and communication that takes place between people. This enables them to learn who they are, as well as what role they should adopt.

Goffman's work on stigma explores the rules, rituals and social processes contained within social encounters that lead to a dominant or consensus definition of a social situation. An analysis of the stigma associated with illness, disease and disability relates to much work done on the sociology of deviance, which explores the ways in which some individuals come to be defined as deviant when others do not.

In a health studies context, the acquisition of a deviant identity occurs through a twofold process (Williams 1987: 137). Primary deviance involves the application of a label, such as a medical diagnosis. Often people reject a label or diagnosis that involves a deviant or stigmatising identity in order to protect themselves or their children from a negative social reaction. Social awareness is also challenging primary deviance by using less-judgemental terminology in making diagnoses. This process is most clearly evident in renaming of mental handicaps as learning difficulties. The second part of the process is secondary deviance. This involves a person's own response to the negative reaction engendered by a label. While some will challenge secondary deviance, many will internalise it and come to see themselves in the deviant role or negative social identity.

Williams highlights the extent to which labelling and the

change to the deviant status often involves some sort of 'degrada-tion ceremony' (Williams 1987: 137), which, in relation to health and illness, may be through surgery such as amputation, mas-tectomy or the formation of colostomy. After these events an indi-vidual learns that they are now labelled as an ostomist, amputee or disabled person, all of which mark them as being different from the rest of society. Stigmatising identity may then come to domi-nate the individual's primary social identity or self-identity and become a 'master status' or 'total identity' which is often difficult or impossible to get rid of. A stigma may also be seen as a 'special kind of relationship between an attribute (what you are) and a stereotype (how you are perceived)' (Goffman 1963: 14). It is there-fore a social reaction that spoils an individual's social identity or self-identity; the ways in which society perceives individuals become central to the ways in which they come to see themselves.

Scott (1972) suggests that a stigmatising identity or label carries negative moral connotations. The bearer of the label is frequently viewed as 'morally inferior'. Stigmatising labels are also seen as 'essentialising labels'; they carry implications about the character of the person that extends to all areas of personality (Williams 1987: 140). Thus, physically handicapped people may often wrongly be assumed to be intellectually inferior. Companions may be asked on their behalf 'does he take sugar?', or 'what is her name?'. When a deviant label is applied in this way, the person is frequently 'marked off from the rest of the group and moved to its margins' (Williams 1987: 140). Goffman showed that in society this means that the person with the stigma is seen as 'not quite human' (Goffman 1968: 15). The stigmatising condition is then used to explain her/his social inferiority, and to discriminate, for example, against a person with a mental health problem or a learning difficulty. Goffman also described what he called a 'courtesy stigma' that spreads out in waves from the stigmatised individual to friends and family, through their close association with the stigmatised individual.

The management of a stigmatising identity

Much of Goffman's work was concerned with the ways in which a stigmatising identity is managed, contained or hidden in social cir-cumstances. Crucial to this is the visibility of the stigma (Goffman

1963: 64). Clearly the level of visibility varies with different conditions, for example, a physical handicap may be highly visible, whereas HIV or AIDS may not be visible at all. The more visible a stigmatising condition is, the greater is the possibility that people will know.

Stigmas may also be context dependent, some conditions are more evident in certain contexts. For example, the handicap of a blind person is obvious in a context where vision is important, as opposed to in a concert where hearing would be a key feature.

Also crucial to the stigma is its *obtrusiveness*, or the extent to which the attribute disrupts normal social interaction (Goffman 1963: 66). A person in a wheelchair, for example, is less obtrusive in a situation where people are sitting down, at a dinner or meeting, whereas a person who suffers from deafness may be obtrusive in circumstances where verbal communication is central. A person with diabetes may be obtrusive when rigid requirements about the timing of meals intrude on the 'normal' flexibility of a day. Epilepsy is a condition in which the obtrusiveness of the condition will vary depending on whether the condition is under control.

Similarly Goffman draws a distinction between the 'discredited' and the 'discreditable' individual. In the former case the stigmatising condition is known about before a social encounter; in the latter case it has the potential to become known (Goffman 1963: 14). Individuals may choose information control as a strategy to manage this distinction. For example, some may choose not to disclose discrediting information about themselves and may attempt to 'pass' for normal. Passing may have high personal cost. It may lead to high anxiety levels, due to the risk of others finding out, which may happen at any time. Examples include a worker with epilepsy who does not disclose the condition to her/his employer, or a person with HIV in a new relationship. Similarly, individuals whose stigmatising attribute is not highly visible may pass as normal in many social encounters as the conventional attribute is not usually on view; none the less there may be certain situations when their attribute will become evident. 'Covering', or attempting to reduce the significance of a stigmatising condition, is also a strategy for people with a stigmatising condition. Covering strategies, such as a blind person wearing sunglasses both to reduce the significance of blindness and to cover evidence of disfigurement or unsightliness, attempt to reduce the significance of the stigmatising attribute.

Goffman's application to illness, disease and disability of the social processes involved in the acquisition of a deviant identity is useful for health professionals as they often work closely with stigmatised people, helping them to accept their 'problem' or make a good adjustment to new circumstances or a new body image. Certain health care practices can, however, reinforce a stigmatising identity rather than reduce it. For example, the provision of a prosthesis following mastectomy can create a conflict between the ways in which individuals are encouraged to come to terms with a disfigurement following surgery and the ways in which people are encouraged to hide their disfigurement from society. A breast prosthesis may help the woman feel 'normal' following mastectomy, whilst at the same time helping to reinforce the idea that one-breasted women are not 'normal'. Some patients, following disfiguring surgery or following hair loss after chemotherapy, refuse to hide their differentness. Action such as this may go some way to challenging the social devaluation associated with certain conditions. Nevertheless, whilst society continues to stigmatise individuals who suffer from disfiguring conditions, or have particular disabilities, many will choose to cover or hide them.

Abberley (1993), in his analysis of disabled people, is critical of the ways in which writers such as Goffman have looked at the phenomena of social devaluation and 'shameful difference'. He is critical of the way interactionist perspectives describe people's beliefs rather than explain them. He states that such analyses help to 'justify the abnormality of disabled people by claiming that it is inevitable' (Abberley 1993: 110). Instead he highlights the economic plight of disabled people, that leads to their powerlessness. He argues that abnormality is not due to individual physical impairment, rather it is located in a society that fails to meet the 'normal' needs of impaired people, which may be different from some, but not all, of its citizens. Such needs might include money for assistance with daily activities of living like dressing or bathing, extra heating, individualised clothing or transportation, all of which can create extra hardship for impaired people.

Abberley highlights the extent to which disablement is located in the social construction of normality, and can be influenced by policies, legislation and social practices which create impediments to a greater participation in the society in which people live (Abberley 1993: 114). Such a conceptualisation is closely associated with a social model of health, whereby rigid parameters of normality and abnormality can be broken down and individuals enabled to achieve their potential whatever their levels of physical ability or impairment.

KEY TERMS

Social construction

A major theoretical position in medical sociology which looks at the way in which sociological phenomena (such as health and sickness) are 'constructed', that is created and understood, in the light of prevailing social standards which themselves generally reflect the standards of the dominant groups within society.

CONCLUSION

Once the social sciences questioned the reductionist view of the causes of sickness and death and moved from specific to multiple aetiologies and from biomedical to social models, then the focus of attention shifted to examining the ways in which ill health was a product of social existence. This process contributed to a rebirth of the public health movement which had, in Britain, become somewhat moribund after its brief period of activity in the nineteenth-century era of sanitary reform (see Chapter 3). As noted in the Introduction to this text, the constitution of the World Health Organization (WHO) had already declared in 1948 that health was 'a complete state of physical, mental and social wellbeing, and not merely the absence of disease and infirmity'. This broad social and psychodynamic definition of health was reaffirmed by the WHO Assembly when the 'Health for All By the Year 2000' strategy was proposed in 1978. It implied that only a broad programme of social policies could adequately address health issues.

The social model continues to inspire those involved in formulating health policies on a global level, even if the practical aspects of their policies often revert to the medical model. Coronary heart disease presents an example of a condition which is now the subject of major health prevention work launched within the 'Health For All' strategy. Two interpretations of its 'causation' are possible. Under a strictly biomedical interpretation the disease would be causally identified by clinical pathology, and found within the malfunctioning of the body. According to the social model, to this diagnosis must now be added the multiple aetiology of lifestyle – diet, exercise, personal history. And using the tools of social science the social construction of that lifestyle itself can be addressed, through examination of, for example, the relationship between poverty and health, exposing factors underlying the aetiology and the choices that people make. 'Health' has moved into the community, into health prevention strategies, into an emphasis on taking personal responsibility, and finding personal and social solutions. In this conceptual shift towards a social model there are also a greatly increased number and variety of people involved in health care; it challenges professional omnipotence and seeks greater involvement by people in their own health.

In conclusion, the social sciences find that the concepts of health and disease and illness have a far greater complexity than that suggested by the medical model. Consideration has to be given to the social, cultural, political and economic factors which influence the environment within which good health may be enhanced or hindered. Attention also has to focus on the diverse ways in which people themselves, or institutions, interpret and deal with such matters.

EXERCISES

1 Compare and contrast the biomedical model and social model of health.

2 Consider the extent to which the sick role is applicable to illness encounters of patients or clients you have come into contact with.

3 To what extent might the actions of health professionals to reduce the visibility of a stigmatising condition, for example, through the use of prostheses, reinforce negative connotations or stigma associated with certain conditions?

Guided Reading

The following texts may be useful for further study into some of the areas introduced in this chapter: Parsons (1951) and Goffman (1963) are original texts; Abberley (1993), Williams (1987) and Stainton Rogers (1991) provide useful further discussion.

Part two

Care in action

Chapter 6

Health behaviour and the individual

■ Rosemary Gillespie

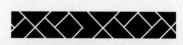

- **The experience of health, illness and disease**

    - lay perceptions

    - explanatory models

    - illness iceberg

- **Health and illness behaviour**

    - triggers

    - health belief model

    - lay referral systems

This chapter will first examine the social and cultural factors that underpin people's understanding of health and illness. Secondly, it will examine the ways in which this might affect their help-seeking behaviour.

Introduction

Previous chapters have explored concepts and definitions of health. In order to work therapeutically with patients or clients, it is also important for health professionals to have a clear understanding of the experience of health, illness and disease, as well as the social processes involved in seeking care. An understanding of the ways in which people understand, interpret and conceptualise their illness experience, can better equip health professionals to communicate with, and therefore help more effectively, people in their care.

The experience of health, illness and disease

This first section will explore the ways in which 'lay' people understand and interpret their experiences of health, illness and disease. Perceptions of 'health' and 'illness' vary considerably across cultures as well as within cultures, with no single explanation for the multiplicity of experiences defined as health, illness and disease.

KEY TERMS

Lay
The shared beliefs or shared culture of the non-professional or non-expert.

Lay perceptions of health, illness and disease

Studies of the interpretation of health, illness and disease in western culture have developed two approaches. First, a traditional approach explores the provision and uptake of services within the biomedical framework. The second approach is a more interpretive exploration of the health and illness experiences of individuals in society. Within this second approach, it is important to understand how people make sense of their wellbeing, disturbance or sickness. The decision to seek professional care, for example, may be only one of a range of alternatives available to people when unwell.

Freidson (1970b) has suggested that lay health beliefs, and perceptions of illness and disease, are, at least in part, the product of medical knowledge. Thus, in a study of middle-class French people, the perceived causes of illness and disease were found to be variations of the ideas contained within medical theories (Herzlich 1973). Stacey has argued that any common ground between lay and professional understanding is not because lay people have internalised the medical model, more that they both draw on common cultural understanding (Stacey 1988: 143).

Writers such as Wendy Stainton Rogers (1991) have challenged the dominant view held by many health professionals, of the superiority of biomedical knowledge, and therefore the legitimacy of its primacy. She outlines the ways in which the dominance of the biomedical approach has often led to the discounting of lay knowledge which may sometimes be seen as a watered-down version of medical knowledge, old wives' tales, superstition or quackery (Stainton Rogers 1991: 3). Thus the complexity of people's experience, she argues, can be seen to constitute alternative, rather than subordinate meanings. She identified eight ways in which people interpret and account for their experiences:

1   The 'body as a machine', closely associated with the medical model where disease is seen as an objective phenomenon with biomedicine as appropriate treatment.
2   The 'body under siege', where the body is as though under threat of attack from germs and diseases, or through the stresses of modern living reaching the body through the mind.
3   The 'inequality of access' account, recognising the value of modern medicine, but suggesting that unfair allocation goes against those who need such services most.
4   The 'cultural critique' of medicine, highlighting a 'post-modern' approach where medical knowledge is seen as a social construct and dominant ideology.

5   The 'health promotion' account, where both collective and personal responsibility for health are recognised.
6   'Robust individualism', where freedom of choice is considered paramount, despite the health effects of particular behaviours, for example, smoking.
7   The 'power of God', where good health is seen to be derived from spiritual wellbeing.
8   The 'willpower' account that emphasises individual responsibility to maintain good health.

Postmodernism

The claim that a fragmentation or dissociation of contemporary society has occurred that has led to the emergence of a new phase in social development, that of postmodernity. This new sociological era casts doubt on scientific rationality. Knowledge therefore becomes contextualised, truth becomes perspective.

Individualism

The emphasis that is placed on individual achievement as opposed to the benefit of community and society as a whole.

Collectivism

The ways in which people act together in order to pursue shared interests or goals to benefit the group or community.

A similar but slightly different categorisation is provided by Chrisman (1977) in an outline of common theories of the causes of illness or 'illness causation', from a review of cross-cultural folk ideas concerning illness:

1   Invasion of the body, through germs or cancer, or through the ingestion of bad food, or other intrusions understood to cause illness.

2　Mechanical factors such as blockage, for example, in the gut or blood vessels.

3　Degeneration, such as the body being run down, or through the accumulation of poisons.

4　Balance, which needed to be maintained through diet, sleep, vitamins to maintain general harmony in the individual or with the environment. This perspective carries specific echoes of the Hygeian approach considered in Chapter 3.

(Chrisman 1977)

Many of these beliefs about health will coexist within societies as well as between them. Some elements will readily be seen to be commensurate with western biomedicine and, as a consequence, biomedicine can be represented as one belief system alongside many others – lay, folk, religious, alternative and complementary medicine. Writers such as Stainton Rogers argue that each should be accorded equal value. The coexistence of competing belief systems is known as medical pluralism.

KEY TERMS

Medical pluralism

The availability of a range of different treatments based on differing belief systems.

Explanatory models

Kleinman (1980) has used the term 'explanatory model' (EM) to illustrate the ways in which specific health and illness episodes are conceptualised by the people experiencing them. Explanatory models may differ cross-culturally, as well as between different social and ethnic groups. In the west, illness causation may be put down to microbes invading or attacking the body, which may be fought with drugs. A Chinese EM may involve an interruption to the flow of one of the six humours, or interruption to the natural cycles of the seasons, causing imbalance between the two oppositional energies, Yin and Yang.

Explanatory model (EM)

A cognitive framework, drawing on a person's belief system, in which an individual makes sense of their illness experience, or health problem. An EM may relate to cause, onset, pathophysiology, course and treatment, and it constitutes the subjective interpretation of an illness episode.

Visual imagery from the social context of people's lives is often a feature of EMs. For example, in the west, military metaphors are used to understand illness and its treatments. The body is often seen to be 'invaded' with an infection that it tries to 'fight'. It might also be seen to be 'run down' in times of stress. Treatments are also frequently explained in this way, for example, illnesses are attacked with drugs, or bombarded with radiation. Similarly, in a religious community, an illness episode may be seen as the will of God; where the supernatural is part of a belief system, illness may be understood to be caused by a neighbour's ill-will. Explanatory models may also differ considerably amongst different social groups. Lay EMs, based in a lay belief framework, may differ considerably from those of health professionals who draw from a biomedical model.

Explanatory models consist of the notions about an illness episode and the associated treatments employed by all those involved in the clinical process, including the patient. If lay EMs differ from professional ones, this may lead to failure of communication between professional and clients. Lay EMs illustrate the significance of the health problem for the sufferer and her/his family and therefore should always be considered. If a doctor's explanation of disease fails to take into account a patient's or client's own beliefs, the outcome may not be therapeutic, the patient may not conform to treatment regimes, and health education opportunities may be lost.

Explanatory models draw on belief systems in response to particular episodes, and enable people to cope with specific health problems (Kleinman 1980: 106). They therefore allow people to make sense of the health and illness events in their lives. The explanatory model framework is useful to illustrate the dynamics of cognitive and communicative interactions in relation to health and health care. It is also a useful tool in the comparison of traditional, alternative, complementary and cross-cultural health belief settings.

The illness iceberg

Studies have shown that only a small proportion of the illness and dysfunctions that exist in the population lead to formal care, most being 'denied, normalised or evaluated as having little importance' (Mechanic 1992). Evidence that illness and dysfunction exist in the population to a far greater extent than that which comes to the attention of the health services has led to knowledge of the existence of an 'illness iceberg' (Hannay 1980). Levels of ill health diagnosed and treated amongst the population appear to represent only the tip of an iceberg, with a greater amount submerged or hidden. For example, in a study of the use of health diaries in women, it was reported that they sought help from the doctor for one out of every forty symptoms (Western and Brown 1989).

The illness iceberg is the result of a considerable accommodation of symptoms, where people learn to live with their health problem, leading to a 'pool' or residue of unrecognised or undiagnosed illness, or unmet need. This pool easily exceeds the amount of illness in medical treatment, at any one time. In order for health problems to come to the attention of the health care services, they have to be recognised by the sufferer and then expressed as demand. If all the ill health in society came to the attention of the health services at once, however, demand would by far outstrip available care. These high and often avoidable levels of unknown sickness, pain and disability that exist in society represent a waste of human, social and economic potential.

Some of the illness that fails to come to the attention of the primary health care services does so because it is treated elsewhere. This may be through self-treatment such as non-prescription medication (Wadsworth *et al.* 1971; Dunnell and Cartwright 1972), or therapies such as acupuncture, homeopathy, osteopathy, hypnosis, massage and aromatherapy, as well as many others.

Which? magazine reported in October 1986 that, in a random sample of people who had used complementary medicine, 42 per cent had consulted an osteopath, 26 per cent a homeopath, 23 per cent acupuncturists, 22 per cent chiropractics and 11 per cent herbalists (Stacey 1988: 158). Such ways of treating illness may be alternative to, and complementary with, biomedicine. This highlights the extent to which an individual's experience of health, illness and disease is not exclusively the extent to which people access primary health care services. Moreover, it is more effectively evaluated by an exploration of what Kleinman (1985) has called 'local health care systems' that include popular, folk and professional services (Scambler 1991: 44).

BOX 6.1

Key types of alternative therapy

Acupuncture – developed in China based on changes in energy that cause symptoms of illness. Acupuncture uses fine needles to one or more parts of the body to stimulate specific points that have a therapeutic effect on distant organs of the body.

Homeopathy – an individualised treatment that uses drugs in small quantities that in a healthy person would produce symptoms similar to those of illness.

Osteopathy – a treatment based on the manipulation of bones and joints of the spine.

Aromatherapy – the therapeutic use of the sense of smell to induce relaxation and promote health.

Chiropractic – the use of manipulation to treat specific disorders such as back pain.

Health and illness behaviour

The first part of this chapter explored the ways in which social and cultural factors can be seen to impact upon individuals' conceptualisation of health, illness and disease. The rest of the chapter will explore how this can affect the ways in which people seek help for health problems: their 'illness behaviour'.

Triggers

Often the decision to seek medical help for illness or symptoms is less straightforward than it might appear. Health problems or symptoms may be recognised as indications of disease, nevertheless medical opinion and treatment are not always immediately sought (Scambler 1991: 40). Irving Zola (1973) highlighted the ways in which individuals frequently tolerated or accommodated symptoms for periods of time before seeking medical help. The health problem or symptoms alone were often insufficient to cause people to go to the doctor; rather, the decision to consult a doctor was related to some select social–psychological circumstance. Zola identified what he called triggers that push people to take action. If triggers were not paid sufficient attention to, for example, during a medical consultation, Zola argued that there was increased risk that the patient would discontinue treatment. In a similar fashion Mechanic (1968) also highlighted ten factors associated with response to illness and seeking medical advice.

The decision to seek care therefore, can be seen to be a very complex issue, involving the interaction of a person's beliefs, values and culture. It is also affected by an individual's perceptions about the personal costs and benefits of seeking care and treatment. All these are taken into account when people decide whether to present themselves at the doctor's surgery, the accident and emergency department or the clinic. In addition, what may be seen as relevant to the patient/client, may not appear relevant to the health professional, which may have important implications for compliance with treatment regimes, and health education opportunities.

The decision to seek care

Five non-physical triggers that prompt patients to seek care (Zola 1973):

1 The occurrence of interpersonal crisis such as bereavement, which may cause a person to become unable to cope with pain or disability.
2 The perceived interference of ill health with social or personal relations.
3 Input from others such as pressure or advice to seek help or care.
4 The perceived threat or interference of the illness in relation to physical or vocational activity.
5 The 'temporalizing of symptomatology': a personal evaluation leading to a decision such as 'if I still feel ill tomorrow, or if it happens again I will see a doctor'.

Ten factors associated with response to illness and seeking medical advice (Mechanic 1968):

1 Visibility and recognisability of symptoms. If a symptom is visible the more likely the individual will be to respond to it.
2 The more serious the symptom is considered to be, the more the chance that it will be responded to.
3 If a symptom causes disruption to the sufferer's life, such as work, family life and social activities, through pain or disability, the more likely it will be responded to.
4 The longer the symptom persists, or the more frequently the symptom occurs, the more likely the person will be to seek medical help.
5 An individual's level of stoicism, or tolerance threshold, will also affect whether or not a person seeks medical advice.
6 The level of personal understanding, knowledge or cultural assumption will also have a determining effect.
7 Psychological processes that distort reality, for example, fear, may cause an individual to delay seeking care.
8 Competing demands on an individual, such as work or child care, which may prevent help seeking.
9 Competing interpretations of symptoms, which are evaluated according to the individual's life situation.
10 The 'opportunity cost' of treatment, in terms of money, time and the effects of such action in terms of embarrassment or stigma.

Health belief models

The health belief model suggests that the extent to which an individual may be ready to take action in relation to her/his health is determined by the person's perceived susceptibility and the consequences of not taking action (Rosenstock 1966; Becker *et al.* 1977). Factors which influence a person's assessment of the benefits of seeking care as well as the costs are seen against the perceived probability that a particular action, such as going to the doctor, will reduce the threat to health. Age, the accessibility of services, general satisfaction with services, clinical practice styles and previous experience are all important factors that structure these decisions and determine whether an individual will engage in particular health behaviour (Morgan *et al.* 1985: 81).

The theoretical underpinning of the health belief model is the idea that those with the appropriate combination of motives and beliefs will engage in behaviour designed to prevent illness, or help restore health. Health professionals might assume that it is always rational for people to report symptoms causing physical problems or anxiety. Action to obtain good health may, however, be only one of a whole list of equally pressing priorities. For example, for the single mother, or for the low-income family, hospitalisation, or time off work, must be seen in terms of the total cost; seeking health care may be uneconomical in some circumstances.

Lay referral systems

Orientations towards illness are firmly established within cultural and social groups and have a considerable influence in the utilisation of health services. Freidson (1970b) outlined the concept of 'lay referral systems' and highlighted the ways people confide in others about health problems before seeking care. These systems affect, first, whether professional care is sought and second, the type of care which is eventually accessed.

Discussions concerning whether to seek professional care often focus, at first, on consultation within families. They then proceed to progressively more distant and authoritative lay people, where a process of 'validation' of symptoms may occur before

KEY TERMS

Lay referral systems

These involve social networks through which individuals pass before seeking professional advice. Essentially they concern the sociocultural attitudes, knowledge and norms of the individual's peer group towards health care.

symptoms are 'sanctioned' and medical advice sought. This process of lay validation may differ markedly from that of health professionals. Frequently, lay culture sanctions illness simply on the basis of whether the symptom deviates from a culturally defined normality, established by everyday experience. Thus, a persistent cough may not be considered abnormal for workers in a coal-mining community and constant tiredness may not be seen as unusual in a group of new parents. Freidson (1970b) suggested that in a subculture considerably different from that of doctors, there exist extended lay referral systems which may actually lower uptake of medical services.

The differential outcomes of lay referral systems with regard to the type of care which is to be accessed are clearly evident in both the Black Report (DHSS 1980) and *The Health Divide* (Health Education Council (1987). These official publications indicated that, considering the greater levels of need in the lower social classes, the uptake of primary health care services of people in these groups failed to match this need. McKinlay (1973) showed, in his study of uptake of ante-natal services in working-class families, that lower levels of uptake of these services were found in groups associated with the existence of an extensive network of lay contact. Similarly, Scambler and Scambler (1981) studied women's perceptions of illness and the effects of lay consultations and found that there were eleven lay consultations for every medical one. Kinship networks appeared to predispose women to consult general practitioners, whilst discussions with friends were shown to have the opposite effect.

CONCLUSION ▬▬▬▬▬▬▬▬▬▬▬▬▬▬▬▬

This chapter has explored some of the complex ways in which individuals conceptualise health, illness and disease. These conceptualisations underpin health and illness behaviour, as well as the processes involved in seeking care. Perceptions of health, illness and disease have been seen to vary across, as well as between, cultures, with much ill health failing to come to the attention of the health care services. The existence of alternative ways of treating illness represents competing rather than subordinate belief systems, and can have significant impact on the health and illness behaviour of individuals and groups.

EXERCISES

1 Find out what complementary and alternative therapies are available for patients or clients in your area, and what proportion of people make use of these services.

2 To what extent might the introduction of market forces into health care services make them more sensitive to individual perception of health, illness and disease?

Guided Reading

To explore further some of the issues raised in this chapter consult Dunnell and Cartwright (1972), Freidson (1970b), Hannay (1980), Kleinman (1980) and Zola (1973).

Chapter 7

The lay–professional encounter

■ Rosemary Gillespie

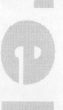

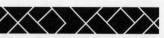

- **Micro-perspectives**

  - clinical-practice style

  - models of doctor–patient relationship

- **Macro-perspectives**

  - social class

  - ethnicity

  - gender

This chapter will examine the relationship between health professionals and individuals and groups in society. It will do this at the micro- or face-to-face societal level and at the macro-societal level.

T HE INTERACTION THAT TAKES PLACE between health care professional and patient/client is of the utmost importance to the delivery of care. It can have significant implications for both the communication that takes place and the outcome of care. Health professionals need an understanding of the complexity, significance and effects of professional–client interactions. There may, for example, be a considerable imbalance of power between doctors and patients/clients through the use of jargon or technical knowledge. This may render the patient particularly vulnerable during a medical encounter. Such encounters often take place in surroundings unfamiliar to the patient, or while they are unclothed, putting them at further disadvantage.

Much of the literature concerning the lay–professional interface relates to doctor–patient interaction, and constitutes an interesting and informative area of research. Much of it is equally relevant to other health professionals who may adopt similar ways of behaving or clinical practice styles. A knowledge of this area of study is also important because health care professionals may find themselves present when an interaction between a doctor and a patient/client takes place. They may be involved in the help and support of patients/clients during such an encounter, or provide continuing support afterwards.

This chapter will explore the nature of the lay–professional interface. It will do so at both the micro-, or face-to-face level, as well as at the macro-societal level, involving large-scale groups or social divisions such as ethnic groups, women and social class.

Micro-perspectives

Meetings between health professionals and clients take place in a variety of settings, for example, in the community, in hospital, in a clinic, during health education activities and elsewhere. Success or failure of the encounter can be significantly influenced by the manner in which it is handled, for example, the amount of information that is exchanged, if indeed any is; whether the patient/client is helped to feel at ease; whether the health professional speaks in language that they can understand; whether the patient/client is given the opportunity to give an account of the problem and listened to. None of this can be taken for granted, and may have significant implications for the outcome of care, and whether the patient complies with a treatment regime or heeds health education advice. Tuckett *et al.* (1985) have shown that two-thirds of patients reporting symptoms did not discuss some of their symptoms with the general practitioner. Failure to report symptoms in this way might have significant implications for doctors' understanding and subsequent diagnosis of patients' problems. This in turn might affect the patient's satisfaction with the service and the outcome of care.

Clinical-practice style

A key factor which may have a significant effect on health outcome is the way in which an interaction between a health professional and a client is managed – the clinical-practice style. Evaluation of clinical-practice style involves an exploration of both the ways people act when they come together, and the ways in which they have, or do not have, common values.

Traditionally, sociologists such as Parsons (1951) and Freidson (1970b) focused attention on understanding the ways in which professionals and patients might seek to exert control during an interaction and thus influence its outcome. More recently, Byrne and Long (1976), in a study of behavioural phenomena between doctors and patients, identified a range of styles of clinical consultation that polarised into those that were doctor-centred and those that were patient-centred. Clinical-practice style was shown to depend on the way the doctor defined the patient's problem; whether it was seen in biomedical terms, or whether the doctor took a broader view of illness in accordance with a social model. Doctor-centred consultations were tightly controlled, used closed questions whereby patients were required to give short answers such as yes or no, for example: 'Do you have a pain here?' This style primarily used the doctor's special skills and knowledge, with patients given little opportunity to discuss their anxieties. The purpose of the interaction was to gather information and reach a medical diagnosis as quickly as possible. Such encounters conformed to a traditional 'paternalistic' medical encounter.

Patient-centred encounters, in contrast, were seen as much less authoritarian, with the use of open-ended questions such as: 'Tell me about these pains.' With this approach the patient was encouraged to give their account of the pain, involving greater participation, and making use of the patient's knowledge and experience. Doctors frequently gave greater attention to the holistic or psychosocial aspects of illness, spending longer with the patient, with time spent listening and reflecting (see Figure 7.1).

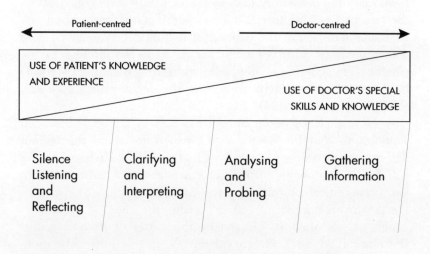

FIGURE 7.1 Patient-centred and doctor-centred encounters in general practice. *Source*: Byrne and Long (1976)

Models of doctor–patient relationships

Morgan *et al.* (1985) have highlighted several models of the doctor–patient relationship which are useful tools for further understanding the nature of the interface between doctors and patients.

Parsons' (1951) consensus model of doctor–patient relationships

This model has already been introduced in Chapter 5 and will be considered only briefly. The relationship between doctor and patient was seen by Parsons as a reciprocal one, closely linked with lay and professional social roles. The doctor was seen as the clinical expert: a person having technical competence (Parsons 1951: 343). Doctor and patient were both thought to have certain rights and obligations attached to their respective social roles as doctor or patient.

see p. 85

Parsons' model of the doctor–patient relationship is one of reciprocity and consensus, despite the inequality that exists between the two parties, due to the doctor's social status, medical knowledge and skills. Thus the patient, in this model, must co-operate with the doctor, and the doctor has to act in the interests of the patient. The consensus implied within this framework reflects the shared value system found in the functionalist approach (Morgan *et al.* 1985: 123).

Nevertheless Parsons' model has been criticised as based on assumptions that the doctor is the expert to whom the patient defers to, and co-operates with. Such assumptions are based on the belief in the rationality of the biomedical model. Freidson (1970b) has been critical of this idealised conceptualisation of the doctor–patient relationship, and especially the medical profession which he described as 'blinded by the glitter of its own status' (Freidson 1986: 381). He considered the relationship to be more of conflicting vested interests than one of mutuality or reciprocity.

Szasz and Hollender's (1956) typology of doctor–patient relationships

Another functionalist analysis of the basic doctor–patient relationship is that of Szasz and Hollender (1956). They see the interaction as a representation embodying the activities of two mutually dependent participants. Consensus between doctor and patient is seen to be 'functional' for society. Their 'typology' highlights three models (see Table 7.1) of interaction between doctor and patient:

- activity–passivity
- guidance– co-operation
- mutual participation

TABLE 7.1 Three basic models of the physician–patient relationship

Model	Physician's Role	Patient's Role	Clinical Application of Model	Prototype of Model
1 Activity–passivity	Does something to patient	Recipient (unable to respond or inert)	Anaesthesia, acute trauma, coma, delirium, etc.	Parent–infant
2 Guidance–co-operation	Tells patient what to do	Co-operator (obeys)	Acute infectious processes, etc.	Parent–child (adolescent)
3 Mutual participation	Helps patient to help himself	Participant in 'partnership' (uses expert help)	Most chronic illnesses, psychoanalysis, etc.	Adult–adult

Source: Szasz and Hollender (1956)

In the first model, activity–passivity, the doctor actively treats the patient, who is passive in receipt of treatment. This is most appropriate for situations when the patient is helpless or in an emergency situation, for example, during surgery, whilst in a coma or during treatment for trauma. Szasz and Hollender make a comparison here with a helpless child and parent. Interaction takes place irrespective of the patient's contribution, and regardless of outcome. The second model, guidance–co-operation, consists of the doctor advising or telling the patient what to do and the patient co-operating with the doctor's advice. This is most appropriate in acute illnesses such as respiratory illness, or when a patient agrees to undergo elective surgery. The patient is expected to defer to the doctor's leadership in the encounter. In the third – mutual-participation – model, the doctor helps the patient to help her- or himself by making use of the expert knowledge of the doctor. This model presupposes that equality between parties is desirable. Examples of this are when the patient is involved in self-care as may be the case for many chronic illnesses or mental health problems.

Stewart and Roter (1989): conflict and control

Both Parsons' and Szasz and Hollender's explanations of doctor–patient interaction are useful but dated models for understanding the lay–professional interface. They do not take into account the possibility that doctors and patients often do not have consensual functional relationships and the conflict that sometimes arises. In contrast, Stewart and Roter (1989) highlight four types of doctor–patient interaction, determined by the varying amount of control employed by both parties, varying from low to high (Figure 7.2). Their model takes into account cultural and demographic factors, as well as stage and type of illness, all of which may be reflected in the doctor–patient relationship.

A paternalistic relationship, where the authority of the physician is unchallenged, depicts the traditional doctor–patient relationship. The level of patient control is low and that of physician high. This corresponds to Parsons' sick role and represents consensus and the traditional form of medical encounter. Mutuality

Patient control	Physician control	
	Low	High
Low	Default	Paternalism
High	Consumerist	Mutuality

FIGURE 7.2 Types of doctor–patient relationship.
Source: Stewart and Roter (1989)

depicts patients having high control whilst physicians also maintain high control. Both parties, in this example, are involved in decision-making, representing a sharing of belief systems and ideas. The consumerist model is where the patient has high control and physician low. The traditional power base is reversed and the patient adopts the more active position in decision-making. Greater consumerism in health care services in the UK, where patients are encouraged to take greater control, may increasingly lead to this type of doctor–patient relationship. This model is also found in a private sector model of the provision of health services where the patient or their representative is a paying customer on whom the doctor is dependent for income. The final type of doctor–patient relationship is that of default. In this example, the patient and doctor both adopt low levels of control over the encounter. This may occur when doctors attempt to involve the patient in decision-making but the patient does not take up this opportunity, perhaps because they do not realise that this is happening or they are used to more traditional, paternalistic types of medical encounter (Morgan 1991).

Different styles of encounter between patients/clients and health professionals may be appropriate in different circumstances. These circumstances may reflect the individual characteristics of patients or their specific health problems. In addition, factors such as patients' understanding of illness and their individual explanatory model, may be of importance in relation to a micro-perspective on the lay–professional encounter.

Macro-perspectives

The nature of the interaction between health professional and patient may also be affected by specific social groupings that the patient may belong to. This section will explore the lay–professional interface in relation to three areas: social class, ethnicity and gender.

Social class

Social class can have a significant impact on the health professional–client interaction. Studies such as the Black Report see pp. 199–202

(DHSS 1980) and *The Health Divide* (Health Education Council 1987) have shown that people in the lower social classes experience greater levels of ill health and early death than their higher-status counterparts. Social class also appears to affect the quality of health care received at the hands of the health services and during encounters with health professionals.

KEY TERMS

Social class

A large-scale system of stratification dependent on economic and occupational differences amongst the population. It distinguishes groups who share certain common factors such as work, resources and spending patterns. Occupational stratification such as the Registrar General's (RG) social classification primarily concentrates on those who are economically active and live in families with a male head of household. It is less useful in the measurement of women, the unemployed, retired people and other groups for whom work is not the organising principle of their lives.

Blaxter (1984) has demonstrated that specialist referrals are highest in Social Class I, and lowest in Social Class V, despite those in the lower social groupings experiencing greater health problems. In addition, Cartwright and O'Brien (1976) showed that working-class patients have shorter consultations with general practitioners and receive less information concerning their health problems than middle-class patients in the same practice. Pendleton and Bochner (1980) indicated that patients from the higher social classes received more explanations voluntarily than did those from lower social classes. A study by Bucquet *et al.* (1985) into GP home visits in London found that families in Social Class I had the highest proportion of home visits while middle-class parents of children in hospital appear to be given more information about their children than their poorer counterparts (Earthrowl and Stacey 1977).

Ethnicity

Ethnicity has also been shown to affect the professional–client interaction. Britain is increasingly a multi-cultural society and, as such, its health care services should reflect multi-cultural health needs. Historically the National Health Service and the health professionals who work within it have been seen to reflect the priorities of the indigenous population at the expense of other members of society (Rowden 1990). Racism and discrimination have been shown to exist in the service and their effects are seen in both patient care and the lay–professional interface (Renn 1987).

BOX 7.1

Britain has increasingly become a multi-cultural society. The regular Labour Force Survey estimated in 1987 that a total minority working-age population was 1,600,000, or 4.7 per cent of a total population of 33,740,000.

It may be that some individuals may choose to discriminate against others due to their own prejudices. In other cases discriminatory behaviour may be learnt through social or cultural norms or through *professional socialisation*. Often, however, people may not know that their attitudes, action or lack of knowledge may harm others. Institutional racism or discrimination is often unintentional at the individual level, for example, traditional *ethnocentric* and bureaucratic practices are often inflexible and not geared to the modern, multi-cultural nature of a community. Practices and regulations often disadvantage people who do not fit the 'Caucasian mould' where, for example, 'pink, healthy skin' is considered the norm.

Racism and discrimination in health services and ethnocentric work practices take limited account of differing health needs and beliefs or the social and cultural construction of illness by differing ethnic groups. The result of this may be that the health needs of groups within the population are not met and consumers

KEY TERMS

Professional socialisation

The process by which people selectively acquire the values, attitudes, interests, skills, knowledge and culture current in the groups of which they are or seek to become a member.

of care may not be satisfied with the service. This will cause patients/clients to feel marginalised; consequently they may not comply with treatment regimes or attend for screening. Health care and health promotion opportunities may be lost. Similarly, problems may be encountered by black and minority ethnic health care workers who suffer racism at the hands of patients.

KEY TERMS

Ethnocentrism

'The tendency to look at other cultures through the eyes of one's own culture, and misrepresent them' (Giddens 1989:739).

Contact with the health care services and particularly hospitalisation, can present considerable problems for individuals from ethnic minority groups. Communication difficulties can be frightening if interpreters are not available, particularly, for example, in the middle of the night or during an emergency. Provision for dietary needs and preferences are also at times inadequate. In addition, services for the particular needs may be difficult to access: some diseases disproportionately affect members of certain minority ethnic groups. Poor access to female medical practitioners for women from groups who require such access for cultural and religious reasons can also cause further difficulties.

Gender

Women constitute both the largest group of health care users, particularly in the areas of reproduction and mental illness, and the majority of providers of health care services (Doyal 1979; Stacey 1988; Hockey 1993). Yet, medicine is seen by many to be one of the areas where structural inequalities which discriminate against women are reproduced. Second-wave feminists have developed a critique of the doctor–patient relationship, with particular emphasis on medicine as a patriarchal institution fundamental to the oppression of women.

see p. 71

The feminist critique has shown the ways in which patriarchal western medicine has been of historical and primary significance in underpinning women's unequal social position (Ehrenreich and English 1976; Oakley 1993). This has been shown to be evident at both the individual level through face-to-face encounters with the male-dominated medical profession and at the macro-level through medical endorsement of patriarchal ideology. Medical power over women can be seen to be particularly evident through control over women's sexuality, contraception and reproduction.

Foster (1989) has highlighted four main strands to the feminist critique of the dominant doctor–patient relationship. First, medical definitions or diagnoses of women's problems are often based on subjective assertions about women's natural state and social role, rather than scientific 'facts'. Examples of this can be seen in Scully and Bart's (1978) critique of the ways in which women have been depicted in gynaecology textbooks. Second, medical advice to women can frequently be seen to be based on dominant male views about women's natural role, such as caring and dependency. The extent to which this is deliberately perpetrated by patriarchal medicine as a weapon to maintain women's subordination, and the extent to which it is genuine advice based on some male doctors' own socialised views about women, remains unresolved, even within feminism. Third, Foster cites the ways in which some doctors exert control through medical advice or treatment of individual patients for what they see as the sake of society as a whole, for example, the sterilisation of certain patients for the 'good of society'. Such action may conflict with the good of individual women. Lastly, Foster draws attention to the hostile reaction of some within the medical profession towards women who have attempted to challenge medical control over their health and health care. She cites documentation in medical notes warning other practitioners about such women and making derogatory remarks about them.

CONCLUSION

The interaction that takes place between health professional and patient or client can have a significant impact on both satisfaction with, and outcome of, care. This is increasingly evident as patients become more aware of their health needs and rights. It also has considerable implications for the increasing part played by health professionals in preventive medicine, health promotion and health education. In a more consumerist, market-oriented health-provider environment, health professionals will increasingly need to pay attention to ways of improving the effectiveness of their encounters with patients and clients.

EXERCISES

1 Discuss the extent to which you have observed an appropriate and an inappropriate clinical-practice style in a lay–professional encounter.

2 Find out what services are available in your area to cater for the specific needs of different ethnic groups.

3 Critically evaluate the extent to which the 'Patient's Charter' may empower women to overcome what the feminist critique has termed 'patriarchal medicine'.

Guided Reading

The following titles provide further development of the areas and issues raised in this chapter: Byrne and Long (1976), Foster (1989), Freidson (1970b), Morgan (1991), Scully and Bart (1978) and Stewart and Roter (1989).

Chapter 8

Institutions, individuals and professional power

■ Martin Giddey

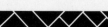

AIM

This chapter examines health care provision placing a particular emphasis on critiques of institutional elements of provision and the professionalisation strategies of health care providers.

U SING INSTITUTIONS AS ITS STARTING POINT, this chapter explores social scientific perspectives which can provide valuable insights into the nature, organisation and functioning of health care provision and health practitioners. Historical and contemporary views are both deployed and issues relevant to patients, professionals and managers are considered. Following a brief introduction to health care provision the chapter consists of two sections. The first (major) section is concerned with institutions and the individual and the second section is concerned with institutions and professional power.

Health care provision

Hospitals are central to the range of health service provision within developed societies. In the United Kingdom, numbers of in-patient beds have increased throughout the nineteenth century and most of the twentieth century. In the last two decades of this century, in-patient bed numbers have declined. This decline is a consequence of three trends:

1   The closure or partial run-down of long-stay hospitals for the mentally ill, people with learning disabilities and frail elderly people.
2   The greater use of residential or nursing home care, rather than hospital care, for people with long-term dependency needs.
3   An increasing emphasis on primary health care, community care and alternatives to in-patient hospitalisation in both the acute- and continuing-care sectors of health need.

Notwithstanding these trends, hospitals continue to be a major resource for health care and are the best known of health care institutions. They are also important because they provide settings in which many trainee health professionals gain clinical training and experience.

Primary health care services are provided from a community base such as a health centre, by family practitioners (GPs), community nurses, health visitors, community midwives and others. These health professionals are often the first point of contact between prospective patients and the health services and, when necessary, they will refer an individual on to hospitals, nursing homes, hospices and residential care homes; these latter institutions are examples of *secondary care services*.

It is useful to make a distinction between *short-stay institutions*, such as district general hospitals, and *long-stay institutions*, such as nursing homes. As a consequence of funding arrangements required by the 1990 NHS and Community Care Act, distinctions are also frequently made between institutions which respond to health need, such as hospices, and those which respond to social need, such as residential care homes.

see p. 235

Institutions and the individual

Originally, the word 'hospital' was used to describe an institution which cared for frail, elderly people and it was their frailty rather than sickness which qualified them for admission. Such 'hospitals' were often funded by charitable endowments and managed by the Church. Institutions which cared for the sick were known as 'infirmaries'. As Chapter 3 suggested, the economic and demographic impact of the Industrial Revolution produced conditions in which the creation of institutions was seen as the answer to pressing social needs and problems. Growing urbanisation and industrialisation in the eighteenth and nineteenth centuries were attended by the construction of hospitals for the physically sick, lunatic asylums, orphanages, workhouses and larger prisons. There was thus a functional separation creating different sorts of hospital institution; as Stacey (1988) puts it: 'Voluntary hospitals treated the deserving poor, Poor Law hospitals the paupers (i.e. the undeserving poor); asylums separated the insane and the isolation hospitals the infectious.'

There are competing explanations for why the growth in variety, number and size of institutions was so prominent at this time. In identifying social reform and philanthropy as key formative influences in the creation of asylums, Kathleen Jones (1972) proposes humanitarianism as the imperative which led to the rise of the institutions. Her conclusion can equally be applied to the physically ill. Growing concern amongst the 'genteel classes' about the plight of people with mental health problems in workhouses was galvanised by social reformers such as Lord Ashley Cooper (later Earl of Shaftesbury). The solution to the problem of unregulated care was seen to lie in the creation of a comprehensive system of asylums run by the State. By means of a series of parliamentary measures throughout the nineteenth century, just such a system was created in Britain.

KEY TERMS

Humanitarianism

A philosophy which emphasises individual and collective responsibility for the general betterment of humankind, particularly for those regarded as 'less fortunate'.

Concern about institutional regulation was paralleled by concern about the squalid and unhygienic conditions which prevailed in the workhouse infirmaries. Lobbying by the Poor Law Board, some members of the medical profession and philanthropists finally achieved an administrative separation of sick people and people with mental health problems from the workhouses. In 1867 the Metropolitan Asylums Board was established and this body assumed responsibility for the management of hospitals for fever cases, those suffering from smallpox and for lunatics. The significance of administratively aggregating these three categories of medical problems lay in the perceived need for segregated care and treatment.

More critical historians, such as Michel Foucault and Andrew Scull have rejected these kinds of explanation. Foucault has been an important contributor to the debate and has written extensively about the origins and political functions of institutions, including hospitals (1973) and mental institutions (1967). It is difficult to summarise concisely Foucault's wide-ranging arguments, but he was much concerned with the political necessity to segregate those sections of the population perceived as 'un-productive' – including the sick and those with mental health problems or learning difficulties – within the developing capitalist economies of the eighteenth, nineteenth and twentieth centuries. Commentators such as Midelfort (1980) and Rothman (1983) have criticised this view as over-generalised and insufficiently linked to the facts of social and economic development.

Whilst Andrew Scull (1992) concedes that humanitarianism may have characterised the intentions of the social reformers of the eighteenth and nineteenth centuries, he argues that intentions are of little importance in themselves. It is outcomes which matter. What had been created was a new apparatus for social control. This apparatus is seen as but one component of a broad process by which the capitalist state secured the containment, control and disempowerment of 'socially deviant' elements within society. Essentially this is a Marxist analysis which is concerned with a materialist conception of history. Social developments, like mass incarceration within institutions, can be explained by economic influences linked to conflicts between classes within society.

It is clear that by the end of the nineteenth century a nationwide system of asylums and hospitals had been created in the USA, Britain and many other European countries and their colonies. Whilst the hospitals and the asylums shared some characteristics, it was the latter which were to prove most problematic. They housed both 'lunatics' (people with mental health problems) and 'idiots' (people with learning disabilities) and little attempt was made to differentiate the needs of these two very different human groups. Contained within the same institutions were people suffering from neurological disorders, including epilepsy and dementia, and a variety of other individuals whose behaviour had prompted sharp moral disapproval and social rejection. Extra-marital sex (by women), homosexuality and masturbation (by both sexes) had been categorised as types of 'moral insanity', which could provide a pretext for admission to the institution. The incarceration of this latter group is an obvious example of the use of institutions for the purpose of social control, rather than for benevolent care and protection.

A large proportion of the nineteenth-century institutions have persisted well into the closing stages of the twentieth century and a major debate about their future has emerged. This debate arises from a broad consensus about the inappropriate and potentially damaging effects of institutional care. Towards the middle of the twentieth century, when many of the Victorian institutions had been in existence for around a hundred years, systematic critiques of institutionalisation began to emerge.

KEY TERMS

Institutionalisation

The long-term incarceration of individuals, whether compulsorily, coercively or voluntarily, for the purposes of treatment, care or social control. Generally carries negative connotations.

The academic disciplines from which these critiques were drawn were varied and included social historians, mental health professionals and social scientists. In reviewing these works Jones and Fowles (1984) concluded that, notwithstanding important differences, there was an underlying theme about the negative aspects of institutions which was common to each. This theme had five aspects:

- loss of liberty
- social stigma
- loss of autonomy
- depersonalisation
- low material standards

Amongst these critiques, the work of Erving Goffman (1991) (see Chapter 5) broke new ground in the sociological understanding of institutions. Whilst many other writers had viewed institutions from the outside, emphasising their social context and the perceptions of staff, Goffman's view was very much from within, examining in great detail the experience of inmates. He made

---

detailed observations of contact between inmates themselves and between inmates and the staff of the institution and suggested that these interactions symbolised power relationships, status differences and unstated expectations. He argued that what he termed 'the institutional underlife' assumed an importance greater than the formal procedures and policies of the institution. He also coined the phrase 'total institution'. Whilst clearly no institution is totally disconnected from life outside, the use of this phrase does convey something of the flavour of the dominating and all-pervasive nature of the institution in the world of the inmate.

KEY TERMS

Institutional underlife
The informal and unofficial behaviours of both staff and inmates within institutions, by means of which people attempt to survive the system and meet their personal needs.

Total institution
A place of residence and work where a number of like-situated individuals, cut off from the wider society for an appreciable period of time, together lead an enclosed, formally administered round of life.

Further critiques of institutional care from within psychiatry emerged during the 1960s and 1970s. These became known as the 'Anti-Psychiatry Movement'. A prominent figure within this movement is Thomas Szasz, who is a trained psychiatrist and psychoanalyst working in the USA. As a libertarian, Szasz views both institutional care and psychiatric treatment as inherently repressive and ethically unacceptable (Szasz 1975). Szasz sees institutions reinforcing the dominance of the medical profession and reflecting the exercise of self-interested power rather than serving a benevolent interest in the welfare of patients.

Before concluding this section, two further influences which have tended to challenge the value of institutional care should be noted. The first of these goes beyond the notion that institutional care may have damaging effects upon individuals. It concerns the idea that by their very nature, 'total institutions' are susceptible to corruption, mismanagement and dangerous care practices. The majority of these problems are low-level, though significant, and are often the result of staff becoming socialised within the prevailing culture of the institution; becoming sucked into routinised, traditional and often uncaring and unevaluated practices. More worrying evidence to support this idea seemed to emerge, particularly during the late 1960s and 1970s in Britain, when a series of scandals of one sort or another within long-stay hospitals was given much prominence in the press. These scandals have been well documented by Martin (1984), and the impact of their reporting has certainly been to undermine public confidence in institutional provisions for those with chronic health problems and other long-term dependency needs. There have also been many accounts by service users which have individually documented personal examples of inappropriate care and institutional malpractice, and that by Vivien Lindow (1993) is a particularly useful example. Her experience of institutional care was that it was often coercive, the manipulation and pressurising of patients to consent to treatment was commonplace and real freedom of choice about care was rarely available.

The second challenge to the institution comes from new therapeutic philosophies such as normalisation and social role valorisation. These have had a considerable impact upon traditional modes of institutional care. The origins of these philosophies lie in pioneering work in the institutional care of people with disabilities in Denmark, but the leading exponent is a Canadian worker, Wolf Wolfensberger (1972). Underpinning them is the belief that the consumers of health care should have the same life choices and opportunities as any other citizen. The ways in which users of health care services may be different from others should be valued, rather than seen as evidence of deviance from assumed norms. Normalisation, and to a lesser extent social role valorisation, have had their greatest impact in the field of learning disability but their influence has also extended to the fields of mental health, physical disability and to the care of frail elderly people. Normalisation is also important within the context of contemporary social policy, since it is one of the fundamental principles on which Britain's community care strategy as described in the White Paper *Caring for People* (DHSS 1989) is based.

KEY TERMS

Normalisation

A therapeutic philosophy which, when applied to institutional or residential care, emphasises individual client/patient choice and the importance of simulating 'homelike' environments.

Institutions and professional power

Almost all institutions, whatever their size, are characterised by bureaucratic structures. These are created to implement the formal rules which are used to regulate internal policies, procedures and practices and which control the interface between the institution and the world beyond its boundaries. Max Weber (1978), originally writing earlier this century, constructed an ideal type of bureaucracy by which he meant bureaucracy in its purest form, and suggested that this would have a number of key characteristics:

1   A bureaucracy has a pyramidal structure representing a hierarchy of authority, in which people control the activities of those at the level beneath them, from top to bottom throughout the organisation.
2   Written rules govern the conduct of officials at all levels. The higher the office, the more likely it is that many rules will need to be considered and interpreted flexibly.
3   Full-time, salaried officials are appointed to a specific position in the hierarchy, and their careers will advance within the organisation according to capability and seniority.
4   There is a clear separation between the tasks of officials within the organisation, and their life outside work.
5   No members of the organisation own the material resources

which they use at work. According to Weber, bureaucracies separate workers from control of the means of production.

A modern hospital seems to match Weber's description of the ideal type fairly closely. For example, it is possible to identify a number of hierarchies, such as those associated with a particular profession like medicine or nursing, and those associated with management. Interestingly, recent reforms of the UK National Health Service have tended to flatten professional hierarchies and to extend those concerned with management.

see p. 193

Morgan *et al.* (1985) have indicated that there are limits to the application of Weber's ideal type to hospitals because 'many hospital personnel are members of a profession which is organised in a different way to a bureaucracy, and in particular is characterised by professional autonomy and non-bureaucratic relationships'. Thus, whilst it is useful to understand the institutional structure of hospitals in terms of bureaucracy, the way in which they actually function will depend to a significant degree on how professional power is exercised by health workers.

Professions and professional power

The ways in which an occupation may be defined as a profession are contentious and problematic. A long-established approach to this problem is that of trait theory. Application of this theory involves comparing the characteristics of a particular occupation to those of other occupations such as medicine or the law, which have traditionally been accepted as professions. The extent to which such characteristics are comparable or equivalent determines whether that occupation is seen as a profession, a semi-profession or a non-profession. Hugman (1991) describes how this theory identifies nursing, social work and the remedial professions as 'semi-professions', principally because they lack a discreet scientific knowledge base and tend to emphasise skills rather than knowledge.

In examining the dominance of health professions within an institutional context, Freidson (1970a) argues that *autonomy* is the key concept: the professional should be self-directing in his/her work. He proposes three characteristics of professional autonomy:

1   Legal or political privilege which prevents the encroachment of other professions. The means by which such privilege is secured is 'licensure' or registration by the state of those who have completed an approved training. Doctors, for example, are qualified and licensed by law to prescribe controlled drugs.

2   The control of a specialised body of knowledge and skills by means of training in an exclusively segregated training school. Such exclusivity facilitates licensure or registration but, importantly, it tends to deflect criticism from others who have not undertaken the same training. For example, radiographers are the specific professional group trained in the use of diagnostic imaging equipment.

3   The existence of a code of ethics with which the professional is expected to comply, the purpose of which is to persuade the general public that the occupation can be trusted. In the UK the continuing professional practice of registered nurses, midwives and health visitors is contingent upon observing a Code of Professional Conduct (UKCC 1984).

A different view of professionalism within health care is discussed by Tuckett (1982) who suggests that *socialisation* is a process central to the attainment of professional status. A new recruit is exposed to the predominant norms and values of an occupational group, often, as discussed earlier in this chapter, within an institutional setting, and gradually absorbs and internalises these until they characterise her/his operational style within the organisation. The predominant norms and values of a profession are maintained informally by group pressure to conform, and this is conceived of as a form of social control.

One of the features of the behaviour of professionals within institutions is territoriality. Each professional discipline is concerned to demarcate the extent and limits of its roles and responsibilities. Rationales for these demarcations are derived from training, qualifications, experience and clinical functions which are exclusive or monopolistic. Whilst these demarcations may be commendable for their clarity, they may also be rigid in a way that makes it difficult for professionals to adapt to changing organisational demands. Extended hierarchies can make intra-professional and inter-professional communication slow and inefficient.

Over the last two decades or so, attempts have been made to

ameliorate both these problems through the introduction of flattened professional hierarchies and the creation of multi-disciplinary teams. Following the introduction of general management to the UK National Health Service in the mid-1980s (see Chapters 10 and 11) the exercise of professional power has been significantly mediated by what has become known as the new managerialism. The general managers of health care services occupy a central position within institutional bureaucracies. Their goals and values are not underpinned by autonomy (as described by Freidson (1970a) above) but are influenced by efficiency targets, market requirements and central political control. Whilst there may be considerable common ground between health professionals and general managers, some tension and conflict between these two groups is inevitable.

A further question which arises from the introduction of general management is whether or not health service institutions have become more or less bureaucratic as a result. The intention of the NHS Management Enquiry (Griffiths 1983) was certainly to re-focus the responsibilities of health workers towards clinical roles and away from time-consuming bureaucratic tasks. However, in requiring a mass of clinical data to inform complex management information systems, general management may paradoxically have increased the bureaucratic demands made upon health workers.

CONCLUSION

It is clear that institutions have been central to Britain's health service provisions for the past two hundred years and will continue to be so for the foreseeable future. An emphasis within social policy upon community care, a mixed economy of welfare and market-based resource allocation are certainly changing the nature of health institutions and the roles of professionals and other workers who are deployed within them. The fundamental purpose of institutions in providing care for dependent and vulnerable individuals cannot confidently be viewed as separate and distinct from their broader political and ideological function of social control. The bureaucratic structures and procedures of institutions will continue to provide an arena within which the fluid nature of professional power exists in dynamic tension with managerialism and the objectives of government.

EXERCISES

1 Which aspects of current health and welfare practice can be considered 'institutionalised'? Consider this question from the perspectives of both staff and patients/clients.

2 Identify a local health service with which you are familiar and discuss the ways in which it may fulfil functions of social control, both directly and indirectly.

3 In what ways might the management of a residential care home reproduce the institutionalising effects of much larger state institutions?

4 Consider a particular health profession and identify the extent and limits of its autonomy. In what ways have these parameters changed over time, and why?

Guided Reading

Goffman (1961) is a seminal work, highly influential within social science, which amply documents the problems with mental health institutions and institutional care. Cohen and Scull (1983) provide a multi-authored text giving detailed theoretical discussion and analysis of a variety of issues relevant to institutional care and control. More general perspectives on institutions and institutional care are provided by Morgan *et al.* (1985) who are also particularly helpful in discussing professional power. Freidson (1986) provides a critical and theoretical text which effectively analyses and extends current debates on the sociological understanding of professions, including health professions.

Part three

Policy and the provision of care

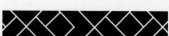

Chapter 9

The founding of the NHS

- Ian Kendall

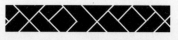

- Key principles of the NHS

- From voluntary health care institutions to a national health service

- Political parties, pressure groups and health services

- Cost containment

- Organisational problems

This chapter provides an introduction to the development of health services in the UK from the first half of the nineteenth century to the second half of the twentieth century including the establishment of the NHS. It will indicate some of the factors that may be seen to have influenced these developments. Through the use of particular examples it will illustrate the extent to which there is an important historical dimension to contemporary issues of cost containment, community care and the organisation of health services.

T HIS CHAPTER TRACES the historical background to the establishment of the National Health Service (NHS) in Britain and the first forty years of its operation. During this period the relative roles of voluntary institutions and state institutions were significantly changed in Britain and other industrial societies. These changes can be linked to changing concepts of health care and the impact of industrialisation and associated demographic changes on society.

see p. 58

see p. 18

KEY TERMS

Voluntary institutions

Organisations which are formally self-governing and independent from the state – although they may be in receipt of some government funding. They are not profit-making organisations and may have the legal status of a charity from which they may derive financial benefits (e.g. exemption from certain forms of taxation).

State institutions

Organisations which are formally linked with and accountable in some way to local or central government.

This chapter will illustrate the importance of political factors in influencing the development of health services. These factors include political ideology, political parties and pressure groups. In particular, it will be apparent that the organisational details of the growing state intervention in health care in Britain were much influenced by the power and interests of one particular pressure group – the medical profession. Finally, the chapter will show that many current 'health service problems' have a historical dimension. These 'problems' may not be identical in the past and the present but there are similarities.

KEY TERMS

Political ideology

A particular set of reasonably consistent beliefs and ideas often associated with particular individuals or groups (including political parties); typically political ideologies will include assumptions about 'how society should be organised' including a view about the appropriate role for the state (see *laissez-faire* and collectivist ideologies as examples).

Political parties

In the UK this refers to organisations that compete for votes at elections in order to be the governing party within central and local government (contrast with pressure groups).

Pressure groups

This refers to organisations which seek to influence the Government but not to become the Government (contrast with political parties).

National Health Service : key principles

The National Health Service was established in Britain in 1948, following the passing of the NHS Act, 1946. There were a number of characteristics associated with this new service. First, it was intended to be a free health service. This did not mean that patients would not pay for the service. It meant that they would not pay to *use* it – the resources to finance the service coming from various taxes levied by the government – for example, income tax and National Insurance contributions.

Second, it was intended to be a universalist service. This meant that everyone was entitled to use the service when they needed it. Deciding when people needed service would be partly a reflection of their own initiative (e.g. consulting a general practitioner, going to a hospital accident and emergency department). However, access to significant (and expensive) parts of the service – e.g. specialist hospital services – would involve an initial consultation with a general medical practitioner who would take responsibility for requesting diagnostic tests on behalf of the patient (e.g. blood tests) and referring patients to specialist hospital services.

KEY TERMS

Universalist service

A service which all members of the population are entitled to use given certain circumstances (e.g. they are ill, they are aged between 5 and 16 years). In the UK the NHS, primary and secondary education are clearly universalist services. This may be contrasted with services that are only available to people with low incomes.

Third, the service was intended to be comprehensive. The aim was to cover all aspects of health care – medical, nursing and other specialist services; hospital and community services; mental health and physical health problems; personal and public health services; curative and preventive services. Finally, the service was intended to be of an optimum standard rather than a minimum standard.

An optimum standard, comprehensive, universal health service free at the time of utilisation implied a significant degree of state intervention in health care. However whilst some features of the new National Health Service were quite distinctive at its inception – particularly being a free, universalist health service – they were not unique in terms of health service developments in Britain or in other countries.

Before the National Health Service

For much of the nineteenth century one particular political ideology, often referred to as '*laissez-faire*', was particularly influential. *Laissez-faire* ideology identified a very limited role for state intervention in economic and social affairs; it was well represented by the Poor Law legislation of 1834 by which the intention was to establish and maintain minimal state intervention in health and welfare. Help for destitute individuals, including the sick, was to be found only in an institution – the workhouse – and only the destitute would seek out such help because the workhouse was to be made deliberately unpleasant. Living conditions in the workhouse were intended to be worse than those of the lowest paid worker living outside the workhouse.

KEY TERMS

> **Laissez-faire ideology**
> The belief that economic growth and the general welfare of society would be most effectively promoted by minimising state interference in economic and social affairs (including matters of health and health care).

Voluntary institutions and health care

If it was intended that the state should have a limited involvement in the provision of health care in nineteenth-century Britain, then there were voluntary institutions which appeared well placed to provide health care instead of the state. Throughout Europe, including Britain, there was a voluntary hospital tradition of providing free care to the poorer sections of the community (Abel-Smith 1976: Ch.1). This was partly attributable to the charitable origins and aims of these institutions, but was also linked to the position of the most prestigious as institutions for teaching and research: 'interesting cases' for teaching and research were as likely to be found amongst the poor as the rich.

Another European trend was the development of working-class voluntary institutions involved in health care. In Britain these were the Friendly Societies. Most of these Friendly Societies provided medical benefit – principally the payment of sickness benefit and payments for the services of general practitioners under contract to provide medical services to their members.

Between them the voluntary hospitals and the Friendly Societies appeared to have considerable potential to meet the health care needs of society. Yet they were both limited. Voluntary hospital provision was limited by two factors. First, the range and scope of private practice, which provided the main source of remuneration for the hospital doctors, concentrated these hospitals in the more affluent and densely populated parts of the country. Second, their focus on the more 'interesting cases' meant that a wide range of health care needs were left unmet by these institutions. As a result there were far more 'sick paupers' in the care of the Poor Law authorities than there were poor patients in the care of the voluntary hospitals (Pinker 1966: Ch.10).

The range and scope of Friendly Society provision was limited by the level and security of people's income. Although they were working-class institutions, regular membership was only feasible for those working-class men in skilled occupations (Gilbert 1966: 166). For those who could not afford Friendly Society membership there were the voluntary hospitals, but for those with 'less-interesting' conditions there was only the provision of the Poor Law authorities.

Industrialisation, urbanisation and health care

One challenge to the *laissez-faire* ideology of minimal state intervention embodied in the Poor Law was 'the public health problem' and the accompanying activities of the sanitary reformers. see p. 23 Although it was developed very slowly, and at first with very limited effectiveness, public health legislation was placed on the statute books (Brand 1965: Ch.1). It seemed that only controls and regulations exercised through central and local government could do something to ameliorate the living conditions and associated health problems in what was becoming a much larger and largely urban population.

These health problems were not only becoming more significant, but typically their victims were excluded from the voluntary hospitals. There was only one place for them to go – the workhouse. The Poor Law authorities thus began to resemble health authorities, in part at least, as a consequence of the sheer size of the nineteenth-century health problem – although the health care they provided was of a very variable, and frequently rudimentary quality. By the end of the nineteenth century it was evident that the health care problems of an industrial, urban society would require more than minimal state intervention in health and social care. What was needed appeared to be some sort of state-provided public and personal health service.

Political parties, pressure groups and social insurance

Significant extensions in state-provided health services were to take place when the Liberal government was in power after 1905. This government was not committed to the *laissez-faire* ideology but to the view that it was appropriate and beneficial for governments to intervene to influence the economy and society in general. This ideology has been labelled as 'collectivist'.

KEY TERMS

Collectivist ideology

The belief in the desirability and benefits of state intervention in economic matters and of the state provision of public services such as health care.

The health care changes in this period extended local government involvement in matters of health and introduced the concept of social insurance. The Education (Administrative Provision) Act of 1907 authorised the introduction of school medical inspections (not a school medical service). However, by 1914 the majority of local education authorities were also providing a school medical service to deal with the volume of ill health detected through the system of inspections. In the same year that local government acquired the powers to develop school medical services, the development of health visiting services was facilitated under the Notification of Births Act, 1907.

A system of social insurance was introduced by Part One of the National Insurance Act, 1911. On the basis of National Insurance contributions by themselves and their employers, all manual workers and other workers with incomes under £160 per annum became entitled to a limited cash benefit in sickness, to the services of a GP and to a pharmaceutical benefit. This was known as the system of National Health Insurance – although it was not national, as it excluded men in non-manual occupations earning over the income limit, most women and all children. Furthermore, it was not a health service, as hospital care was largely excluded.

The establishment of National Health Insurance (NHI) in the UK proved controversial with the Liberal government drawn into conflict with interest groups whose financial circumstances were adversely affected by the introduction of a state-regulated system of health insurance. These groups included the Friendly Societies, the doctors and the industrial insurance companies. In the end a compromise was reached in which the administrative arrangements for NHI were so ordered as to allow a role for industrial insurance companies in managing the scheme alongside the Friendly Societies and by devising a level of remuneration and form of employment (as self-employed practitioners) which accommodated the professional sensibilities of the doctors (Gilbert 1966: Ch.6).

These administrative arrangements had a long-term significance in so far as the self-employed independent contractor status of GPs has been retained in the NHS ever since. In addition the development of a state-funded and regulated GP service reinforced the existing referral system when some voluntary hospitals refused to treat patients unless they were referred by their NHI doctors; by so doing it reinforced the role of GPs as key 'gatekeepers' to the rest of the British health care system.

Pressure groups, in the form of Friendly Societies, industrial insurance companies and the medical profession, clearly had an influence on the important organisational details of these health care changes. Political parties may also have played a part in this period of reform since all the changes took place when the Liberal party was in power. The next dramatic extension of state intervention in health care in Britain – the setting up of the NHS – would come when another 'left of centre' political party (the Labour party) was in power.

The emerging case for a National Health Service

By 1936 local authorities had an obligation to provide or at least finance an adequate midwifery service and the power to provide a home help service. This was in addition to their other powers and obligations to employ health visitors and to provide a school health service as well as their long-standing public health responsibilities. Local government was also a major provider of hospital care, including most mental hospitals. Of particular significance was the Local Government Act, 1929, which abolished the Poor Law authorities and transferred all their powers, duties, buildings, personnel and paupers to county councils and county boroughs. Given the limitations of the voluntary hospital system, this included a large number of 'sick paupers' and the hospitals and hospital staff who cared for them.

Despite these developments there were calls for more radical reforms. Health services were widely perceived as both inefficient and insufficient to meet contemporary needs. A partial National Health Insurance scheme that excluded children, non-earning wives, the self-employed, many old people and higher-paid employees, operated alongside other services whose scope and effectiveness depended on the wealth of each area and the political initiative of different local authorities. There was clear evidence see p. 202 of what was later to be labelled 'the inverse-care law'. Those parts of the country with the worst health status appeared to have the worst health services – at least when measured by numbers of doctors and hospital beds (Titmuss 1963: 143–4, 214).

War and the health services

In 1939 a major war began in Europe in which Britain was one of the main protagonists (Second World War, 1939–45). It might have been anticipated that this major event would preclude further discussion and any action on the issue of health care reform. However, the perceived inefficiencies of the hospital sector of the health services were of immediate concern to those planning measures to cope with what was feared would be significant civilian air-raid casualties (Abel-Smith 1964: 425). The solution to the haphazard and extremely variable quality of existing hospital services was their temporary nationalisation in the form of the Emergency Medical Services and in October 1941 the Ministry of Health announced that the Government was committed to establishing a comprehensive hospital service after the war (Honigsbaum 1989: 28).

The following year saw the publication of the Beveridge Report. The report was primarily about social security (i.e. family allowances, pensions, unemployment benefit), but it appeared to capture the public imagination with its evocative references to the five giants of disease, idleness, ignorance, squalor, want. These were to be attacked by policies for health, employment, education and housing as well as social security. It was as part of this broader battle against these giants that Beveridge identified a crucial role for a universal, comprehensive health service: 'medical treatment covering all requirements for all citizens will be covered by a national health service ... treatment will be provided for all persons capable of profiting by it' (Beveridge Report 1942: 11). The following year (1943) the Government announced that it welcomed the conception of a reorganised and comprehensive health service which would cover the people as a whole and include institutional treatment.

Political parties, pressure groups and the National Health Service

There was considerable public support for the proposals in the Beveridge Report and especially for the National Health Service (Calder 1969: 609). None the less there were major controversies concerning the administrative and financial details of how the new National Health Service was to be organised. Given the important pre-war role played by local government, the initial proposals for the NHS envisaged a key role for local government. But this provoked considerable opposition from the medical profession. Many general practitioners were anxious to maintain the self-employed independent contractor status established with the introduction of National Health Insurance. Both GPs and hospital doctors wished to avoid becoming salaried employees of local government. This was perceived as a threat to 'clinical freedom'.

The results of this professional opposition can be seen in the organisational structure eventually assumed by the new National Health Service when it came into operation in 1948. This was called the 'tripartite structure' in which the NHS was organised around three main elements which were administratively and financially separate from one another (see Figure 9.1). First, all the hospitals – local government and voluntary – were nationalised and virtually all of them were placed under regional hospital boards and hospital management committees. Secondly, family practitioner services were to be administered by executive councils and GPs retained their self-employed status. Thirdly, the role of local government in health care was limited to a range of community health services. In addition the most prestigious institutions – the teaching hospitals – were given a special status and considerable organisational autonomy in the new structure.

The National Health Service: the first forty years

In the period leading up to the establishment of the NHS the hope was expressed that a national health service could be developed that would 'diminish disease by prevention and cure' (Beveridge Report 1942: 162). The resulting lower demand on health care resources held out the possibility of stable or even decreasing costs for the new service. The reality was one of higher demand and increasing costs. The outcome was predictable. Within twenty-one months the first cash-limit was introduced into the NHS; charges were introduced for dentures in 1951 and for spectacles and prescription charges in 1952. It was apparent that containing the costs of the new NHS was firmly on the political agenda (Abel-Smith 1990: 12).

The post-war period saw a continuing growth in new forms of medical intervention and the development of new therapeutic methods – most involved additional expenditure. It also saw a continuation of demographic trends in which the proportion of the

Special Family Hospitals	Teaching Hospitals	Non-teaching Hospitals	Community Health Services	The Practitioner Services
		330 hospital management committees	Maternity and child welfare; domiciliary midwifery; health visiting; home nursing; home helps; prevention of illness; mental health and welfare work; vaccination and immunisation; ambulances	Doctors, dentists, drugs and appliances, ophthalmic services
	Board of governors	15 regional hospital boards	175 local health authorities (county, county borough and district councils)	134 executive councils

FIGURE 9.1   The tripartite structure of the NHS, 1948–74

population aged 65 years and 75 years and over increased. People in these age groups place higher demands on modern health services. In addition the publicity surrounding advances in medical technology probably contributed to rising expectations about what the service could deliver. In combination, these factors increased the potential volume of treatable illness confronting the NHS. Successive governments found themselves confronting a situation in which additional expenditure was necessary merely to enable the service to maintain its current level of provision.

see pp. 36–7

Planning the NHS

One means of getting a more efficient health service was through planning. There was a notable lack of planning in the pre-war health services and the wartime experience had indicated the potential for national and regional planning as a means of remedying perceived deficiencies in service provision.

Peacetime planning was to prove more difficult at least in part for political reasons. These included the political concern with cost containment already identified – a relatively short-term focus on limiting expenditure is not always compatible with the longer-term perspective required for planning. Planning may also be seen as at least partially a victim of professional power and influence. For example, a planned reduction in spatial inequalities in health services (the 'inverse care law') required a change in the distribution of doctors between different parts of the country but the medical profession was reluctant to agree to proposals that placed significant restrictions on where doctors could work.

The first major exercise in national health service planning did not come until the publication of the Hospital Plan for England and Wales (Ministry of Health 1962) in 1962. But it was a hospital plan not a health service plan. The plans for the health and welfare services of local authorities in England and Wales (Ministry of Health 1963) included community health care but showed little evidence of a co-ordinated approach to both hospital and community health services. Since these rival plans were the products of different parts of the 'tripartite' organisational structure they could be taken as further evidence of the limitations of this structure – especially for the development of effective health service planning.

Reorganising the NHS

Under the 'tripartite' structure the NHS was administered by more than 500 separate administrative units, based inside and outside local government, and servicing areas which were not necessarily geographically coterminous one with another. Effective use of hospital resources was clearly dependent on effective use of community health services enabling the earlier discharge of patients who no longer needed 24 hours a day in-patient care. But the 'tripartite' structure separated hospital and community health services. Effective use of community health resources was clearly dependent on effective co-operation between medical and nursing services enabling general practitioners to work as a team with, for example, district nurses. But the 'tripartite' structure separated community-based medical practitioners (GPs) from the community-based nurses (domiciliary midwives, district nurses and health visitors working for local authority health departments).

In 1968 the Ministry of Health published the first Green Paper on NHS reorganisation initiating a five-year period of debate and discussion culminating in the NHS Reorganization Act, 1973 and the introduction of a new organisational structure in 1974 (see Figure 9.2). This new structure was soon to attract as much criticism as the previous system for being over-bureaucratic and top-heavy with managerial hierarchies. It was also seen as affording rather limited gains in terms of organisational change. One part of the previous organisational division between hospital and community care went with the virtual elimination of local government health responsibilities and the transfer of community health hospital services to area and regional health authorities. But the administration of GPs remained largely separate via family practitioner committees.

Furthermore, in 1971 a separate reorganisation of personal social services within local government had created social services

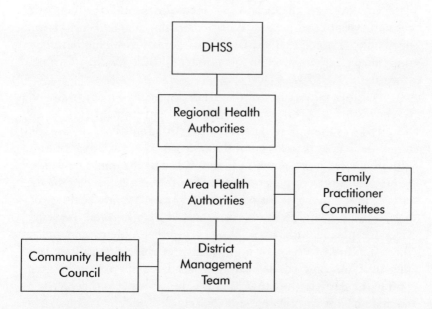

FIGURE 9.2 The 1974 NHS reorganisation. *Source: Jones and Moon, 1987*

departments with major responsibilities for developing community-based services for elderly people and people with mental health problems and learning disabilities. The result was that policies for community care were still hampered by what was to become known as the health/social care divide. Health care services (e.g. home nursing and day hospitals) were to remain the responsibility of the NHS; social care services (e.g. home helps and day centres) were to remain the responsibility of local authority social services departments. These arrangements would be the subject of several critical reports in the 1980s culminating in a major reform of the organisational and financial basis of community care (see Chapter 14).

Priorities in the NHS

The pursuit of a more equitable allocation of health care resources was one of the more clearly stated goals of the service (Klein 1983: 25). The key inequalities concerned the allocation of, access to and the utilisation of the resources and facilities of the NHS. The service's inheritance was of profound spatial inequalities with a set of associated inequalities linked to social class. Chapter 12 provides detailed coverage of social-class inequalities and the equivocal response of governments to doing something about them. Here it need only be noted that spatial inequalities in resourcing have been the subject of attention in government NHS funding formulae since the mid-1970s.

Another inheritance of the NHS, especially linked to the different histories of the voluntary and local government (Poor Law) hospitals was the different provision for different types of care, different groups of patient and different sorts of need. Some of these differences are represented in Figure 9.3. The diagram can be used to identify contrasting sectors of the health services. It suggests that community-based care for people with chronic mental health problems will be relatively less well resourced than hospital-based services for people with acute physical health problems and indeed there appeared to be growing evidence of these inequalities from the late 1960s onwards as a series of scandals and crises drew attention particularly to the provision for elderly people and people with mental health problems and learning disabilities. The label 'Cinderella services' was attached to this part of the NHS. The particular focus for concern was the long-stay institutions which seemed to be providing poor quality care in settings that were increasingly felt to be expensive, unnecessary and stigmatising. Attempts to redress the balance of resources in favour of the 'Cinderella areas' effectively began with the publication of a consultative document on priorities for health and personal social services in England (DHSS 1976).

see p. 87

Low prestige/priority	High prestige/priority
mental health	physical health
community-based	hospital-based
caring	curing
preventive	curative
health promotion	medical intervention
chronic health	acute health
terminal care	life-saving interventions
disability	disease

FIGURE 9.3 'Cinderella services'

CONCLUSION

The establishment of the NHS in 1948 did not represent the beginning of significant state intervention in health care in the UK. State intervention in health care has a long history; it can be traced back at least as far as the Poor Law and public health legislation of the nineteenth century. The scope of this intervention was significantly extended before 1948, most dramatically by the Liberal government with the introduction of National Health Insurance and more gradually by the acquisition of duties and powers by local government. However the establishment of the National Health Service by the post-war Labour government did signify a commitment to important new principles – a comprehensive, optimum-standard service available on a universalist basis largely free at the point of consumption.

The development of the NHS provides clear evidence of the enduring significance of particular issues. The detailed organisational arrangements of health services have proved to be consistently controversial. The administrative arrangements eventually introduced were clearly a political compromise. In both instances the medical profession was active as a pressure group seeking to influence government decisions. The particular concern of the profession concerning professional autonomy expressed itself in support for the independent self-employed contractor status for GPs and minimising the role of local government in the provision of health services. This concern obviously pre-dates the establishment of the NHS and remained a significant factor when the service was reorganised in 1974 when GPs again retained their distinctive organisational status and there was a further dramatic diminution of local government involvement in health care.

These political compromises over organisational structures proved significant in exacerbating divisions between hospital-based and community-based care and limiting the potential of a national health service to be effectively planned. However, the pursuit of effective planning was also inhibited by a concern with cost containment. But the factors that have made cost containment an issue for the NHS and other health care systems in industrial societies are not new. Increased life expectancy was already creating financial problems for the Friendly Societies before the introduction of National Health Insurance and escalating costs were posing severe problems for the voluntary hospitals before their integration into the NHS.

EXERCISES

1 National Health Insurance was one of the social policy reforms of the Liberal government (1905–18). The National Health Service was one of the social policy reforms of the Labour government (1945–51). Identify the other major social policy reforms introduced by these governments.

2 List the main similarities between the events associated with introduction of National Health Insurance and those associated with the establishment of the National Health Service.

3 Identify those problems for the National Health Service which can be identified as being present before the service was established.

Guided Reading

The background to the establishment of the NHS can be placed in a broader historical context by reading Jones (1991). A detailed review of the years leading up to the establishment of the NHS can be found in Honigsbaum (1989). The first forty years of the NHS are well covered in Allsop (1984), Leathard (1990) and Klein (1989a).

Chapter 10

Reforming the NHS

- Ian Kendall

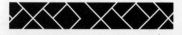

- Health care policy under post-1979 Conservatism

- The continuing case for the NHS

- Organisational and management change

- Spending on health care

AIM

This chapter provides an introduction to the more recent history of the NHS in Britain with particular reference to the effects of the change of government in 1979. It will illustrate the continuing significance of certain issues. These include the concerns about the costs of the NHS and the adequacy of its financial, organisational and management arrangements.

T HIS CHAPTER TRACES THE BACKGROUND to recent
changes in health policy including the major White Paper
(*Working for Patients*, DoH 1989) which introduced a number of
initiatives including the internal market, NHS trusts and fundholding GPs. The Government which introduced these changes
seemed to be committed to a political ideology similar to the nineteenth-century ideology of *laissez-faire*; this commitment appeared
to pose a major threat to the key principles of the NHS. In the
event the NHS survived and its basic principles were given
resounding public support in *Working for Patients*.

see p. 146

Changing government and changing ideology

Since the NHS was established in 1948 there have been several
changes in the political party which formed the Government of the
day. The post-war Labour government (1945–51) which introduced
many social policy reforms was succeeded by a lengthy period
of Conservative government (1951–64). Between 1964 and 1970
the Labour party was in power again. They began the process
which led to the 1974 reorganisation of the NHS (see Chapter 9),
a reorganisation which was completed by a Conservative government (1970–4) and then put into effect by another Labour
government (1974–9). Partly in response to the criticisms of
the 1974 NHS reorganisation, the 1974–9 Labour government
established a Royal Commission on the NHS. When the Royal
Commission report was published the governing party had changed
again.

Changes in government have been associated with significant
changes in social policies, including policies for health care. Major
changes – the introduction of National Health Insurance and the
NHS – were associated with reformist, 'left of centre' governments
(see Chapter 9). However, it has been suggested that alternate
periods of Labour and Conservative government in post-Second

World War Britain did not herald major changes in policy. The period has been categorised as one of 'post-war consensus'.

KEY TERMS

Post-war consensus

An assumption that changes in the political party in power in the UK between 1951 and 1979 involved limited changes in social and economic policies as there was considerable agreement between them regarding key elements of these policies. For example, they both supported the welfare state and government intervention in the management of the economy.

The election of the Conservative government with Mrs Thatcher as Prime Minister has been identified as the end of the 'post-war consensus'. This is because the new government was identified with a particular political ideology sometimes labelled the 'New Right' or 'radical right'. The term 'Thatcherism' has also been used – named obviously after the Prime Minister. Two important themes have been identified with the Conservative government elected in 1979. First, there was a belief in the virtues of the market – that the market is the best mechanism for producing and distributing resources. In particular the market is seen as more efficient and more responsive to people's needs than the state provision. Secondly, there was an emphasis on individualism – the belief that the individual is to be seen as self-reliant and responsible for her or his own actions (Savage and Robins 1990: 5–6).

Although these themes have been identified with the 'New Right' they can be seen as very similar to the *laissez-faire* ideology that was particularly influential at the beginning of the nineteenth century. A belief in the virtues of the market and individualism implies a very limited role for state intervention in economic and social affairs. Commitment to this political ideology would seem to raise serious questions about the future of the NHS. Despite the idea of a 'post-war consensus' there had always been politicians and commentators who had questioned the concept of a National Health Service on the basis that health care needs of the population could best be met by the operation of a private market system rather than a government-financed and regulated health care system. Now there was a government in power which seemed to share this view.

The Royal Commission and the cost of the NHS

The first major government publication on health care in 1979 was that of the Royal Commission which had been set up by the previous Labour government (Royal Commission on the NHS 1979). The Commission endorsed the general criticism of the 1974 reorganisation but in other respects lent considerable support to the concept of a national health service and to the basic priorities of the service. The Commission's brief had included the examination of the possibility of a greater reliance on insurance and charges as a means of financing the NHS. It rejected both, emphasising a point which was to be made with considerable force over the next decade – that by comparison with the health care systems of other advanced industrial societies, the NHS was remarkably cheap and by implication probably quite efficient.

What is revealed by international comparisons is that the problem of controlling and containing escalating health care costs is not confined to the UK. This is unsurprising since the factors linked to escalating costs – demographic trends, medical advances and rising expectations – are associated with industrialisation and increasing affluence. On the other hand, conventional economic analysis might lead to the assumption that the problems of cost containment would be particularly difficult for the British NHS. Its principles of a comprehensive, optimum-standard service available to the whole population seem to imply higher rather than lower expenditures on health care. If we add to this a service which is largely free at the point of consumption we appear to be in a situation where there are no reasons for potential patients to moderate their demands because of cost. Indeed, it might be suggested that individuals will abuse and exploit a service to which no costs are attached.

In the event, as the Royal Commission concluded, the UK spends significantly less of its resources on health care than a number of other countries leading to the paradoxical conclusion that a universal, open access, free service making little or no use of conventional market mechanisms is much better at containing costs than more market-oriented systems. In particular the NHS has a tradition of low administrative and management costs by comparison not only with the market-oriented system in the USA but also the schemes of other European countries like France. The North American experience is one particularly interesting element in the evidence which casts doubt on the wisdom of a more overtly private market solution to health care problems. Since 1971 Canada's switch to a universal and largely government-financed system has led to a levelling off of health care costs by comparison with the increasingly competitive and commercial system in the USA where costs have continued to rise dramatically (Ham 1990).

The relatively low costs of the NHS may be attributable to a number of factors. At least part of this success may be the service's traditional role as the major purchaser of drugs, equipment and the services of health care professionals. If health care professionals in the UK have few alternative sources of employment to the NHS, then the service is well placed to keep wage and salary rates lower than they would be if a number of health care providers were competing for what might be scarce professional skills. In addition, whilst the degree of planning in the NHS was more modest and less effective than had been hoped by some advocates of a national health service, it was sufficient to eliminate the over-provision and duplication of resources associated with other health care systems. Finally, a note should be made of the system of paying doctors employed in the NHS. In particular, the British system has made significantly less use of fee-for-service systems especially for its hospital doctors. Such systems tend to encourage excessive medical intervention involving, for example, higher incidence of surgery and what may be regarded as wasteful use of diagnostic tests (Abel-Smith 1976: 62–3).

see p. 154

The secret 1981 review

Despite the Royal Commission's endorsement of the NHS and its basic principles, the Government commissioned its own review of the financing of health care. This still officially unpublished 1981 review was intended to reduce the extent to which health services are financed by the taxpayer and involved examining a number of alternatives including an almost total switch to private spending (Carrier and Kendall 1990: 89). It seems likely that the Government was deterred from publishing the report because of a growing awareness of the popularity of the NHS amongst the general public. Certainly official government policy made no mention of a dramatic retreat from the concept of a National Health Service. The future of the NHS seemed reasonably secure and previous commitments to reduce inequalities in resource allocations to regions and to the 'Cinderella areas' were continued. On the other hand, the foreword to the Black Report (DHSS 1980) noted that the policy recommendations contained in that report could not be considered because they were too expensive. This suggested that, whilst the Government had abandoned the notion of eliminating the burden of taxation associated with the provision of the NHS, it was very keen to moderate that burden in various respects. One means of doing this would be to make the service more efficient.

Reorganising the reorganisation

The initial attempt to make a more efficient service took a relatively conventional approach. The organisational structure established in 1974 was subject to a further reorganisation (DHSS 1979). This was unsurprising given the substantial volume of criticism directed at the 1974 reorganisation; much of this criticism had been endorsed by the Royal Commission. The result was the abandonment of any attempt to maintain a geographical relationship between local government and health authorities and the adoption of a simple structure based on districts and regions. The new administrative structure came into effect in 1982. Subsequently it was confirmed that the family practitioner committees (FPCs) would be reconstituted as separate health authorities in their own right (Figure 10.1).

This process of organisational change was less contentious than those associated with the establishment of the NHS and the changes introduced in 1974. This may reflect the degree of consensus about the need for change but also the absence of the ideas most likely to generate conflict – changing the independent

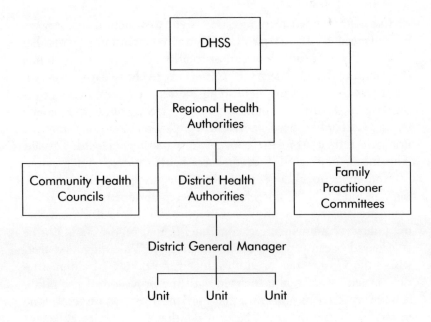

FIGURE 10.1 The reorganised British National Health Service, 1982.
Source: Jones and Moon, 1987

contractor status of GPs or enhancing the role of local government in health service provision. The most controversial aspect of the new organisational structure was the extent to which, after many years of debate and considerable investment of resources, another 'tripartite' organisational structure had been established with a major division between social care (the responsibility of local authority social services departments) and health care (responsibility of the NHS), with the latter divided into two by the continuing separate organisational and budgetary arrangements for GPs.

The potential to develop effective policies for community care for elderly people, people with mental health problems and people with learning disabilities would continue to be restricted by these continuing administrative, budgetary and professional divisions between health and social care. The failure of the 1974 and 1982 reorganisations in this respect, was to be the subject of a series of critical reports in the 1980s. These criticisms and the burgeoning social security budget for private sector nursing and residential care were key factors in drawing the Government into a set of

see p. 230

community care reforms that clearly parallel the changes introduced in the NHS.

Reorganising the reorganisation suggested that the Government did not intend to follow through the full implications of the 'radical right' ideology and undertake a dramatic retreat from state involvement in health care. It did, however, take steps to lessen the burden on the taxpayers of a universalist health service and these steps included more than conventional organisational reforms. They took four forms:

1   A less free service. Perhaps the most obvious means by which the burden on the taxpayer could be diminished was by increasing the burden on the service user. Of course charges were not a new element in the 'free' NHS but, none the less, new charges were introduced (e.g. for eye tests) and well-established charges (e.g. dental and prescription charges) were increased by significantly more than the rate of inflation. However, the NHS still remains one of the health care systems that makes least use of direct service-user charges as a source of finance.

2   A role for non-state health care. The NHS would cost less if people turned to non-state institutions for their health and social care, and the Government sought to encourage and emphasise the virtues of these alternatives to the NHS. Steps were taken to reduce significantly the role of the NHS in the provision of ophthalmic services. The White Paper on services for elderly people contained an unequivocal statement that the advancement of community care would rely less on public provision and more on the community itself (DHSS 1981) and the voluntary sector found itself drawn back into mainstream provision in areas such as day care. Previous attempts by Labour governments to limit pay beds in NHS hospitals and control private hospital development were both abandoned. Supportive comments were made regarding private hospitals and nursing homes as alternatives to the NHS. The latter received dramatically increased indirect support via the social security budget. This had the paradoxical effect of increasing government involvement in traditional forms of residential care. The escalating costs of this policy may have been one of the factors influencing the Government's

commitment to reform policies for community care. It was certainly subject to criticism in a report of the Audit Commission (1986).

KEY TERMS

Pay beds

Pay beds are provided in NHS hospitals to accommodate private patients under the care of NHS consultants who do not work full time for the NHS. The individual patient or their health insurer is billed for the hospital services provided.

Social security

This term is applied to cash benefits such as pensions, income support and family credit. This has also included payments to contribute towards the costs of elderly people or people with disabilities living in privately run residential care institutions.

3 Cost containment and contracting out. The old theme of cost containment was pursued by requiring health authorities to produce efficiency savings; drug budgets were cash limited; generic prescribing of a limited list of drugs and resource management were introduced. Contracting-out and competitive tendering were also introduced. Ancillary services were the main target. Private sector firms would be given the opportunity to tender for contracts to provide catering, cleaning and laundry services. The theory was that the most efficient contractor would provide the cheapest tender and the NHS would benefit from cheaper and more efficient services. This was seen as an effective way of containing costs and bringing the virtues of private sector management into a large public sector organisation.

4 Managerial changes. The perceived virtues of private sector management were introduced more generally to the NHS through the introduction of general management. This topic

is reviewed in depth in the next chapter. Here it need only be noted that, in 1983, an independent NHS management inquiry headed by Roy Griffiths observed there was a 'lack of a clearly defined general management function throughout the NHS' (DHSS 1983: 11). To remedy this situation they recommended the introduction of a single general manager acting as a chief executive and final decision taker. The Government's commitment to the appointment of general managers regardless of discipline instigated the notion that health care is a business in which managers should manage efficiently using management skills which might be applied with equal effectiveness in other public or private sector organisations.

The Conservative government went into the next General Election (May 1987) seemingly confident that the reforms it had put in place, culminating in the introduction of general management, had provided the basis for a more efficient NHS and that no new major reforms were required. However, there was evidence of pressure building up for further reforms in the NHS before the General Election. In April 1987 it was reported that some teaching hospitals were refusing to accept patients from outside their boundaries without some form of payment from the patient's health authority (Carrier and Kendall 1990: 90).

By September 1987, it was being reported in the press that health authorities might be making their biggest round of ward closures and deferred developments for at least four years. By mid-November, many hundreds of beds had been taken out of service. It was at this rather inauspicious time that the Government published their White Paper on primary care. This proposed more spending on family doctor services, paid for in part by new and higher charges. It included measures to introduce more competition between GPs, tougher monitoring of their work, more preventive and health promotion and more information and consumer choice for patients (DHSS 1987).

The growing perception that the service was in serious financial difficulties was given further confirmation in December when the Presidents of the three senior Royal Colleges – the surgeons, the physicians and the obstetricians and gynaecologists – issued a statement warning that the NHS had 'almost reached breaking point'. This mounting public and professional concern in the latter half of 1987 were certainly major factors in the establishment of a major review of the NHS in early 1988, which would seem to be fairly represented as an exercise in crisis management. Its establishment was announced within eight months of a general election in which the Conservative party's manifesto had contained no indication that such a review would take place and within a fortnight of John Moore (Secretary of State for Social Services) dismissing rumours that any such action was intended.

Working for patients

The process of reviewing the NHS took one year. During that time a substantial number of reports and position papers were published. The situation was also confused by the Government's understandable and plausible claim that spending on the NHS was rising not only in terms of money spent (cash terms) but also in what is called 'real terms' – a situation where expenditure is rising faster than the rate of inflation. These claims, and their concomitant linkage to calls for cost limitation, warrant brief consideration.

The rate of inflation relates to changes in the Retail Price Index (RPI). The RPI is a useful index, but has its limitations, and does not reflect the spending of particular groups in society such as pensioners who spend a disproportionate part of their relatively low incomes on heating. The RPI may thus not be very helpful for judging changes in government expenditure on health care. It is possible to construct an index which does take account of the prices of inputs within the health sector. For most of the 1980s the prices of these inputs were increasing faster than other prices, meaning that the 'real increases' were less than seemed to be the case. In addition it was estimated that it might be necessary to increase NHS expenditure by something like 2 per cent per annum to meet the extra demands of an ageing population, medical advances and service developments. The endpoint of this reasoning is that the increases in cash expenditure on the NHS were substantially less significant than the Conservatives claimed.

Professional concerns about inadequate resources can, of course, always be dismissed as special pleading. Obviously the doctors and nurses will say we should spend more on the NHS.

However, in this case it does seem that the concerns expressed by the Royal Commission had some substance. The NHS may not have needed further organisational changes but it did, in the late 1980s, seem to need more money to meet the demands and expectations of patients, professionals and politicians.

The NHS Review was published as the White Paper *Working for Patients* (Cmd.555) on 31 January 1989. It was billed by the Prime Minister as the most far reaching reform of the NHS in its forty-year history. However some aspects of the White Paper had a familiar ring to them. The Government was convinced that raising the performance of all hospitals and GP practices to that of the best 'can be done only by delegating responsibility as closely as possible to where health care is delivered to the patient – predominantly by the GP and the local hospital' (DoH 1989: 3). This theme of maximum delegation had been advanced by successive governments since the first proposals for reorganising the NHS were published in 1968.

The establishment of self-governing NHS trusts – self-managed units independent of the regional and district health authority hierarchy – is in accord with this principle of maximum delegation. Yet even the concept of the self-governing unit was not entirely new to the NHS, resembling in certain respects the status of the teaching hospitals under the original tripartite structure that operated from 1948 until 1974. The White Paper clearly targeted 'major acute hospitals' for trust status (DoH 1989: 28) and, given the interest of some of these institutions in developing an internal market, one can see key aspects of the reform having their origins in the perceived interests of one of the most traditional sources of power and influence – the senior doctors in the most prestigious hospitals.

Whilst self-governing trusts would move out of direct control by regional and district health authorities, the separate family practitioner authorities were to be incorporated into the regional structure. All the health authorities were to adopt a more managerial approach and automatic local authority representation on district health authorities was to be ended. This can be seen as the end of a process lasting over forty years in which the once central role of local government in health care was to be dramatically diminished and then marginalised. The removal of appointed local councillors from health authorities ended the last tenuous links

175

between the NHS and conventional systems of local democratic accountability. However, since neither service users nor taxpayers had ever been given the opportunity to elect any of the members of previous key health authorities – regional hospital boards, hospital management committees, boards of governors and area health authorities – the diminution of democracy in the NHS afforded by this reform was somewhat modest.

The allocation of resources to regions and districts was to be amended. The previous system took account not only of the populations served but also of the services provided. The resources allocated were intended to compensate those districts containing units drawing patients from catchment areas beyond the district. For centres of regional and national excellence this could be very far afield indeed. The new system would be based on the local population weighted for age and the relative cost of providing services. In future all cross-boundary movements would be accompanied by a movement of funds, rather than the movements being anticipated and to some extent pre-determined in the initial allocation of resources. The money would follow the patient in a much more precise and identifiable manner. Hospitals' financial health thus became inextricably bound up with their ability to attract patients.

The most controversial reform, one inextricably linked to the notion of money following the patient, was the establishment of an internal market in the NHS. The internal market involved the separation of purchasing and providing functions of the NHS. The unitary health service, in which a health authority both planned care and provided it through hospital or community services, was to be abandoned in favour of a functional separation of purchasing – buying health services to satisfy local need – from providing – the day-to-day business of delivering that care. Purchasing agencies, holding a budget to ensure the health of a defined population, identifying health needs, planning ways to satisfy them and ensuring the quality of the service, were to develop contracts with the providers who would, in turn, invoice the purchaser for care. General practitioner services were to be brought into the internal market through direct allocation of budgets on a voluntary basis to larger general practices to enable the buying of certain hospital services. These General Practice Fund Holders (GPFHs) were thus to be, simultaneously, both purchasers and providers of health care.

The publication of the White Paper provoked a number of concerns about the operation of the internal market. Would hospital trusts specialise in areas of greatest 'economic gain' and would the market ensure that these were appropriate to the needs of local communities? Might hospital trusts tend to discharge patients to the community before it would otherwise be appropriate? Would budget-holding GPs have an incentive to get their patients admitted to hospitals as emergencies rather than straightforward referrals? Would people with costly problems of ill health find themselves being treated by reference to the size of a general practitioner's budget and the accessibility of specialist hospital care, rather than by reference to their real care needs?

Inevitably the main question that people wish to pose and seek to answer is whether the NHS will be a better service as a result of the changes introduced following the White Paper. This question remains unanswerable at present. One reason for this is that the Government chose to encourage, rather than require, the adoption of trust and fund-holder status. The first trusts and fund holders constituted a distinctly biased sample. Furthermore, some of the identified benefits – especially of fundholding – may not be sustained if the status is more widely adopted. In addition some considerable time needs to elapse before all hospital and community health services have trust status and all GPs have fundholding status. Meanwhile medical advances, demographic trends and rising expectations continue to have their effects on the demand for and provision of health services. By the end of the century health care in Britain may be radically different from that provided before the White Paper was published. In some respects it may be judged better and in some respects worse than that available before the reforms were implemented. But to what extent any of the changes can be directly attributable to the reforms will be very difficult to judge.

CONCLUSION

In reviewing these more recent developments in health care policies it is important to note the enduring significance of particular issues. The detailed organisational arrangements of health services remained controversial – especially with the introduction of general managers and the internal market. Some of these changes can be represented as a reduction in professional power and influence with control shifting to the new general managers. On the other hand the internal market had the support of some teaching hospitals – always regarded as bastions of consultant power. Furthermore, the professional autonomy and influence of GPs might be enhanced by their assumption of fundholding status. In the period under review political ideology appeared to assume a greater significance than for many years previously. However, the survival of the NHS and the 'crisis-management' background to the major reform were indications that other political factors (e.g. winning votes at elections) played a role in government action and inaction.

The most interesting issue for the immediate future must be the continuing impact of the internal market on the operation of the NHS. Some of the implications of the internal market – competition between provider units for scarce resources – are perceived by Conservative sources to keep down costs. None the less there remains the fundamental question of whether the hoped for efficiency gains from the internal market will outweigh the costs of managing the internal market with its complex contractual relations.

EXERCISES

1 It is expected that each year the National Health Service will require more money than it used in the previous year. List and illustrate those factors which lead the National Health Service to require additional resources every year.

2 Identify the services needed to provide adequate health and community care services for either elderly people or people with mental health problems or people with learning difficulties and construct an organisational chart to illustrate the range of service providers that might be involved.

3 List the main advantages and disadvantages that have been identified with the working of the internal market.

Guided Reading

Coverage of the fortunes of the NHS under the post-1979 Conservative governments is enormous. Simple reviews are provided by Ham (1990: Chapter 2) and Kendall and Moon (1990, 1994). A more extended discussion can be found in Ranade (1994).

Chapter 11

Managing the NHS

- Nancy North

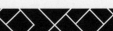

- Consensus management

- Professional power and management

- Public sector management and efficiency

This chapter reviews changes in NHS management styles during the 1980s and considers contemporary approaches to the management of the service.

THIS CHAPTER COMPLEMENTS CHAPTER 10, which provided a recent history of the NHS. The intention in the present chapter is to focus specifically on the issue of management and outline the major changes in NHS management which have occurred in the 1980s. These will be discussed in relation to perceived improvements in management, control of the NHS from the centre and the impact on professional groups, including nursing. Before embarking on this discussion, the chapter will describe briefly the management process leading up to the watershed of the Griffiths Management Inquiry (1983). Griffiths' main recommendations will be discussed, as will the emerging impact of the NHS and Community Care Act, 1990.

The 1970s – consensus management

Periodically during the brief history of the NHS, governments have raised concerns about its efficiency and related to this, whether its organisation and management were appropriate. In 1974 the reorganisation of the NHS formalised *management by consensus*, the idea being that unanimous decisions about local policy would be arrived at after a debate among equals. In addition to regional and area health authorities, district management teams comprising senior hospital doctors, GPs, nurses and NHS administrators, were responsible for administering health services locally. Decisions on how to run the NHS at regional, area and district level were expected to reflect annual and strategic plans. The regular cycle of producing plans became an increasingly cumbersome process as the 1970s progressed.

Consensus management acknowledged the importance of the medical and nursing professions' 'expert' contribution to health care planning. The critiques of medical power and the biomedical model had yet to grip the imagination of politicians. The nursing profession moreover, had been bolstered by the recommendations

see p. 65

of the Salmon Report (Ministry of Health 1966), which proposed a managerial structure for nursing beyond ward sister, up to a hierarchical apex of regional nursing officer.

The underlying assumption of consensus management was that individuals would debate issues and come to a logical conclusion. Inevitably this proved to be too optimistic a view. Close observers of the NHS, and such research studies that exist, indicate the largely political nature of decisions about the allocation of resources and the shape of services within health authorities (Ham 1990; Klein 1989a). A generous interpretation of such political activity would be that the differences of opinion reflect diverse analyses of issues and the means of addressing them. Alternatively, dissent might be considered to be the product of professional syndicalism, each professional group manoeuvring to protect its own interests. The medical profession, as revealed in Chapters 9 and 10, constituted a powerful, if not always homogeneous, group in NHS politics. Salmon and consensus management gave nursing a place in the post-1974 NHS management structure, but nurses were less able to exploit the situation than the medical profession. According to Strong and Robinson: 'The elaborate hierarchy, the lack of any developed sense of professional identity and the initiation into submission from the earliest years meant that nursing was extraordinarily weak in the face of external opposition' (Strong and Robinson 1990: 38).

The Griffiths Management Inquiry

It was not the charge of too much 'politicking' *per se* which ended consensus management, but a growing perception in Whitehall that the style of management it epitomised in the NHS, and indeed in other parts of the public sector, was inadequate. The Conservative governments under Margaret Thatcher were much influenced by the theories of certain academics and politicians, collectively termed the 'New Right'. As well as criticising the extent of state involvement in welfare, these theorists argued that it was inefficient for the state to set up huge bureaucracies (such as the NHS) as providers of welfare. It was alleged that this inefficiency was caused partly by the tendency of those working in welfare services to expand services beyond what was needed, serving no-one's interests but their own in the process. Another criticism offered was that those who worked and managed welfare bureaucracies were buffered from the challenge of competition and so had no incentive to be efficient in what they did, or to respond to the views of those who used the service.

BOX 11.1

The New Right approach to the welfare state

- Bureaucracies, such as the NHS, were unwieldy and inflexible.

- They were inefficient, both in the identification of priorities and the performance of their functions.

- They were insensitive to the needs of clients in structuring their services.

- The professions involved in welfare delivery were self-serving and lacked accountability.

- Overall, the welfare system in the UK encouraged dependency amongst its recipients.

Concern to improve what they saw as an inefficient managerial system, ill adapted to meet the challenge of a dynamic and voracious health care system, prompted the Government to appoint an inquiry team. Roy Griffiths and a small group drawn from management in the public and private sector (Griffiths 1983) were asked to examine whether the NHS's resources were being managed efficiently in order to give value for money. Some of the inquiry's observations were damning:

1   Consensus management produced 'lowest common denominator decisions' and led to long delays.

2   There was little evidence of management objectives being set; of measurement of health outputs or of clinical and economic evaluation of clinical practice.

3   There was no individual ownership of and responsibility for the development, implementation and evaluation of management plans.

4   There was a lack of leadership.

The proposed structure

The Griffiths Report (1983) recommended a streamlined management structure based on the 1982 reform of the NHS and with clear lines of accountability between one layer and the next. General managers, rather than managers in charge of one group of professionals, were to be appointed at unit, district and regional level. Regional general managers (RGMs) were answerable to the Chairman of a proposed NHS Management Board (NHSMB); after the NHS and Community Care Act (1990) this was succeeded by the NHS Management Executive (NHSME).

BOX 11.2

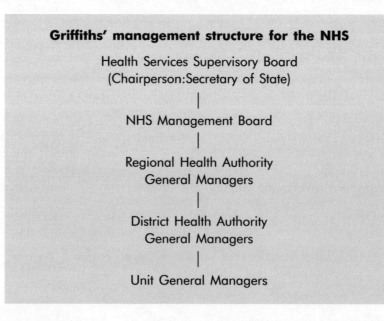

Griffiths' management structure for the NHS

Health Services Supervisory Board
(Chairperson:Secretary of State)
|
NHS Management Board
|
Regional Health Authority
General Managers
|
District Health Authority
General Managers
|
Unit General Managers

In addition to general management responsibilities, managers were to be held responsible for the performance of their district or region against objectives set by the respective supervisory authority. Unit general managers were charged with ensuring budgetary control, a task which paled into insignificance alongside their other responsibility, that of luring the medical profession into the management process. At national level a Health Services Supervisory Board (HSSB), chaired by the Secretary of State, would set out the objectives and overall strategy for the NHS, as well as reviewing its general performance. Accountable to the HSSB, the NHSMB was to be responsible for policy implementation.

Other recommendations

1   General managers were to be subject to sanctions and incentives: performance-related pay, individual performance review and short-term contracts were subsequently introduced.
2   Mechanisms for monitoring the performance of authorities and their managers were urged.
3   The introduction throughout the NHS of the concept of efficiency savings; money was to be saved by working more efficiently.
4   The medical profession were advised to accept the degree of management responsibility appropriate for the use of scarce and costly resources. Budgets held by hospital consultants were proposed.
5   The Government were advised to allow local managers the freedom to manage. Managers were urged to take more notice of consumer opinion when planning services.

The Griffiths Report was accepted by the Government and introduced rapidly throughout the NHS. According to Carrier and Kendall (1986) all Regional General Manager and the majority of District General Manager posts were filled by July 1985.

BOX 11.3

Emphases within the new style of general management

- clear assignment of responsibility for actions

- clear statement of objectives

- emphasis on outcomes rather than processes

- use of private sector provision to increase efficiency

- greater use of rewards and penalties to promote performance

- focus on cautious resource use – e.g. through cutting labour costs – to contain rising costs of health care

Adapted from Hood (1991)

Life after Griffiths – an appraisal

Evaluating the impact of the Griffiths Report is not a simple matter. Griffiths himself felt that it would take a decade before the reforms began to show firm results. The difficulty of evaluating a policy ten years on is that later policies may well have affected its outcome; Griffiths is no exception. During the 1980s the Government required the NHS to make efficiency savings and compared the performance of each district health authority (DHA) with others through the use of nationally collected data known as performance indicators. These and other management tasks handed down from Whitehall created a management agenda in the 1980s from which it is difficult to isolate the particular effects of Griffiths. Furthermore, the development of internal markets and the purchaser–provider split which followed the NHS and Community Care Act, 1990 (see Chapter 10) has muddied the research waters. Fortunately several researchers such as Strong and Robinson (1990), Pollitt *et al.* (1991) and Flynn (1991) completed empirical research in 1986–7, 1983–8 and 1987–8, respectively. Their work, together with the assessments of other academics will be used to evaluate the effects of Griffiths.

According to Strong and Robinson (1990), the business model of management proposed by Griffiths was unable to be fully grafted on to the uncompromising organisation that was the NHS. Even though the performance of managers could be shaped by rewards and penalties, this particular form of behaviour therapy could not be applied to the remainder of NHS staff who remained in fairly secure posts and whose pay was negotiated nationally by powerful unions. However, writing with the benefit of a few extra years' hindsight, Butler suggests that general management changed 'the climate of opinion' and 'laid down the foundations of a management culture of command and obedience' (Butler 1992: 18), a process which has created an increasingly compliant NHS. It is an observation which suggests that, in the passage of time since Strong and Robinson's research, the culture of managerialism has been reinforced.

Managers interviewed in Strong and Robinson's study also recognised the need to change staff attitudes towards 'patients' and to keep a watchful eye on the development of this change in house style. One off-shoot of this concern was the emergence of quality assurance units often headed, according to Klein (1989a), by nurse managers dispossessed by the Griffiths initiative. By contrast Pollitt *et al.* (1991) found a degree of cynicism, with a majority of both nurses and doctors regarding consumer initiatives as cosmetic. Given the retrenchment in health service funding, this was a predictable perception. The work by Pollitt *et al.* also indicated that the nurses they interviewed felt decision-making had speeded up post-Griffiths, whilst district- and unit-level managers were ambivalent over the question. The consultants and senior managers interviewed were the least optimistic. Most managers also felt that the personal accountability of managers had been clarified, though consultants again were the least likely to confirm this.

Flynn (1991), examining management in relation to NHS cutbacks, gave some indication of the increased centralised control of the NHS. He argued that this was produced by three pressures: penalties and incentives, inducing an obedient general management cadre; the threat of penalties being inflicted on overspent authorities; and the appointment of DHA chairpersons by the Secretary of State. He suggested that these pressures resulted in a reluctant acknowledgement by health authority members, managers and the medical profession alike, that there was a need for more financial restraint. Harrison (1988) also suggests evidence supports the view that the managers created following the Griffiths Review were under more pressure to heed government directives and less likely to challenge the centre's policies.

Griffiths and nursing

The toehold that the nursing profession had gained in the NHS managerial hierarchy with Salmon and the 1974 reorganisation, disappeared with the advent of Griffiths. The previously protected positions of nurses (and nursing) at district and regional level were discarded by managers with an eye on sizeable nursing budgets (West 1992). Nurses had to compete for general management positions alongside non-nurses and if successful, carry out functions which more often than not had little to do with nursing services. West suggests that these actions were supported by those consultants 'who had always felt that the only useful nurse was a bedside nurse' (West 1992: 56).

The nursing profession gave a mixed response to this development. Some nurses felt it was important that members of the profession should succeed to senior management posts, so that they could safeguard the interests of clients (and presumably nurses!). Others were less certain, arguing that nurses as general managers would have to surrender loyalty to the profession and conform to a different set of values. It has been recognised that nurses, like the medical profession, are ill prepared to take up posts in general management. More nurses, however, are taking up the opportunity to study management at undergraduate and postgraduate level. The Government has supported this trend by introducing a scheme whereby selected nurses are given grants to undertake further education in management.

Griffiths and the medical profession

Griffiths, like other NHS reports in the past, had recognised the need to involve doctors in management, either by appointing them to general management positions or by giving them responsibility for budgets covering their clinical practice. In effect this made them accountable for the limited resources at their disposal. The notion of clinical autonomy (a physician's right to determine the most appropriate care for her/his client) in the past had prevented any external deciphering, co-ordination or scrutiny of medical practice. However, apart from some isolated cases of medical enthusiasm, the evidence suggests that few doctors were interested in taking up managerial posts.

Doctors also continued to exercise significant clinical autonomy (Hunter 1991a). Although some of the doctors interviewed by Pollitt and his colleagues indicated they had become more cost conscious, Pollitt *et al.* (1991) point out that this feeling could have been a result of the constraints on NHS funding rather than the values of general management. Flynn (1991) argued that financial constraints had created tensions between managers and doctors by bringing the prioritisation of services into sharper focus and threatening established services. The overall impression is thus one of medical intransigence. There was little that management could do other than persuade or manipulate. Other measures were required and in due course were introduced. As one DGM accurately prophesied in the mid-1980s: 'There are ways to control doctors, but they are not available to us yet and they won't be for five years or more' (Strong and Robinson 1990: 162).

BOX 11.4

A district general manager talking about doctors:

'You have to pick them off one by one. . . . For example we've got a very difficult surgeon here. We've been wanting region to discipline him for eighteen months. He refuses to discuss anything with us at all. But he does want new equipment. I said to him, "Fine, there's just one thing. You'll have to sit down and discuss your workload with me."
. . . And, you know, within two days he did it!'

Strong and Robinson (1990: 92)

Management and the internal markets

In an earlier section of this chapter some of the influences of the New Right on Conservative party thinking were identified. Concerns about the inefficiency and profligacy of welfare bureaucracies, such as the NHS, were married to the belief that improvement would be achieved either by using or aping the private sector. The Griffiths model of management was one aspect of this. However, the 'quasi-private' model of management introduced into the NHS, and the strategies associated with it, lacked the important private sector sanction of competition.

KEY TERMS

Clinical directorates

These are sub-units within provider trusts offering a recognisable cluster of clinical services. Usually they consist of several consultants and associated staff and each directorate holds a budget which covers costs. The clinical director, normally a senior consultant, is responsible for ensuring that DHA and GPFH contracts for the directorate's services are complied with.

This deficiency was corrected with the NHS review and the introduction of internal markets (see Chapter 10). In effect the split between DHA and GP fundholding purchasers and service providers has empowered managers in both DHAs and trusts or directly managed units (DMUs). The previously powerful hospital consultants are now further removed from decisions about how DHA monies are to be allocated. In addition the reforms required the doctors to participate in regular audit of their practice. As contracts become more searching and precise, senior doctors have found themselves having to demonstrate that the treatment they provide reflects the most effective, best-cost option.

One initiative introduced to encourage participation in management by doctors and medical awareness of treatment costs was the *clinical directorate*. Other measures, such as changes in consultants' job descriptions and financial rewards for greater involvement in management, also encourage conformity to the changing managerial ethos. In essence, therefore, the current increasing involvement of hospital doctors in NHS management and their growing recognition of their accountability for the resources they use is evidence that the full and effective implementation of Griffiths' recommendations required the catalyst of the NHS reforms.

CONCLUSION

In the twenty or so years since the introduction of consensus management, the NHS has undergone fundamental changes, the full effects of which have not yet emerged. Managers, acting as a type of 'health civil service' have tightened their grip on the NHS. Whereas once they could be described as having a conciliatory approach to the medical profession, the processes initiated by Griffiths and enhanced by the NHS reforms have enabled them, in theory, to adopt a more bullish approach to management. The same period has seen the weakening of professional power in the NHS.

Though never the professional Goliath that was, and arguably still is medicine, nursing's transitory dalliance with health care management was focused on nursing services alone. Its comparatively minor impact on the NHS as a whole must reflect the relative power of nursing and medicine. By the same token the medical profession had more to lose from the more proactive form of management which Griffiths sought to introduce. From the mid-1980s onwards, management honed its skills on a number of tasks required of RHAs and DHAs by central government. The NHS reforms created additional impetus to managerial change, by providing quasi-market conditions and the means of exerting greater control over the hospital consultants.

It is difficult to predict with any certainty whether this process will continue into the next millennium. The increasing numbers of GP fund holders may well affect hospital sector purchasing by gradually diminishing DHA direct control. Trusts, and the consultants who work for them, are likely to contract increasingly with individual fund holders or groups of fund holders (consortia). Whatever form future management incentives take, the process of change is likely to be unremitting.

EXERCISES

1 Jot down what you think were the underlying assumptions about how people behave which were associated with consensus management.

2 Reflecting on the perceived difficulties of consensus management, what improvements would you suggest?

3 Do you think nurses should become involved in senior NHS management? Give reasons for your answer.

Guided reading

Ham (1990) is a well-written book which discusses key elements in the development of managerialism in the NHS. Pollitt *et al.* (1991) offers a valuable insight to the early years of Griffiths. Strong and Robinson (1990) is filled with illuminating quotations from the many managers interviewed and offers a thoughtful and sophisticated analysis of the early impact of Griffiths, including its effects on the nursing profession.

Chapter 12

Health inequalities

- Rosemary Gillespie
- Robin Prior

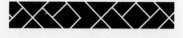

- Social class and health

- Health inequalities

- Policy and inequality

This chapter reviews the evidence and related policy proposals concerned with inequalities in health. It takes as its starting point the findings of the Black Report (DHSS 1980).

O NE OF THE FOUNDING PRINCIPLES of the NHS at its inception in 1948 was *equity*. This meant that the financial see p. 153 worry associated with medical treatment should be removed by the provision of a free service. Despite this, significant differences persist in both the health, and incidence of disease, in the population. This chapter will explore some of the evidence to suggest that, whether individuals or their children are healthy or unhealthy, or whether they die prematurely, is not just a matter of fortune but is linked to one's position in the social hierarchy and is, thus, *structural*.

Social class and health inequality

There is considerable evidence to suggest that in many countries there are differences in health within the population both between different social groups and between different geographical regions (Whitehead 1992). Such differences in health appear to arise as a result of unequal social positions, for example, differing social class, or membership of certain social groups such as ethnicity and gender. They are compounded by geography because people of particular social classes or from specific ethnic groups concentrate in certain locations.

Inequalities in health are important because they highlight the unfavourable health status of certain individuals in society. Whitehead has further indicated that inequalities in health are important because they may be unnecessary and avoidable, and are evidence of unfairness – disproportional suffering between social groups (Whitehead 1992). They also highlight a waste of human economic potential.

The major way in which inequalities in health have been measured in the UK is through comparing levels of mortality and morbidity, for different social classes. Social classes rank occupations in accordance with social status and prestige. They also indicate factors such as income, educational level, behaviour and patterns of consumption, which affect the life chances of individuals within similar social groupings, based on occupation and prestige. Social class is, however, just one of the ways in which social divisions may be measured, others might be gender, ethnicity or locality.

TABLE 12.1 Social class

Class	Category	Example occupations
I	Professional, higher administrative	Lawyer, doctor
II	Intermediate professional and administrative	Manager, teacher, nurse
III (N)	Skilled non-manual	Clerk, police, secretary
III (M)	Skilled manual	Chef, bus driver, baker
IV	Partly skilled	Post worker, farm worker
V	Unskilled	Cleaner, car park attendant

Social class based on occupation is not, however, ideal for measuring inequalities in health. First, in measuring occupation it does not always reflect levels of income or poverty. Second, it is often an inaccurate measure of the social status of certain groups such as retired people and women. Women who are married or live with their fathers may be ascribed the social status of the (male) head of the household, which may bear no relation to their own occupational status, although studies show that it can be a significant predictor (Baxter 1994). Third, disadvantages in relation to health may have more to do with membership of a different social grouping than occupational classification. The unemployed, certain ethnic groups and women, for example, may experience additional health hazards. Social class may therefore act as an indicator of the kinds of experiences and life chances that people might have in common, but it is not an ideal means for the measurement of inequalities in health.

Inequalities : the evidence

The health of individuals is affected by how they live: the kind of work they do; how much money they have and where they live. These experiences relate to unequally distributed life chances that derive from the social and economic roles that people have. It is therefore possible to refer to inequalities of health (rather than just differences) because they appear to be associated with wider social and economic inequalities. Various studies, the most comprehensive of which has been the Black Report (DHSS 1980), have indicated consistent inequalities in health between different occupational groups and between males and females.

The main patterns and trends in health inequalities (DHSS 1980; Whitehead 1987) should be seen in context. As Chapter 1 has shown, during the twentieth century there has been a general fall in mortality and a consequent increase in life expectancy. Whilst the fall in infant mortality has been most noticeable this century, the overall death rate fell more during the last half of the nineteenth century. The main publications on health inequalities suggest that:

see p. 18

1   There is a clear *class gradient in mortality*: the lower the occupational class the higher the mortality tends to be, and vice versa. This gradient is also evident with *infant mortality*, particularly in the case of post-neonatal mortality. Since different occupational classes tend to have different incomes, housing, etc. it follows that there is also a similar association between mortality and these factors. Indeed, if income alone is considered the association with mortality may be even stronger (Wilkinson 1986).

2   Class gradients in mortality vary with the *cause* of death and are generally more marked in adults than children (excepting infants).

3   Patterns of *morbidity* follow similar trends, except that inequalities are lower among adults than for children. Children of manual workers are much more likely to suffer respiratory infections/diseases and be accident victims. Among adults, limiting long-standing illness is twice as likely in the lower occupational classes (Table 12.2). Acute illnesses show a growing link with occupational class as age increases beyond 45 years.

TABLE 12.2 Reported long-standing illness or disability: by socio-economic group, 1989 (GB) (percentages)

Condition group	Professionals	Employers and managers	Intermediate	Skilled manual	Semi-skilled	Unskilled
Musculoskeletal system	10.0	12.6	13.0	15.5	17.1	20.1
Heart and circulatory system	6.4	8.1	8.0	9.4	11.8	12.1
Respiratory system	5.2	5.2	6.8	6.4	7.2	9.6
Digestive system	2.1	3.3	4.0	3.9	4.8	5.0
Nervous system	2.5	2.1	3.1	2.7	2.9	4.4
Eye complaints	1.5	2.2	2.9	2.0	3.0	3.2
Ear complaints	1.9	1.4	1.9	2.7	2.5	3.1
All long-standing illness	29.1	32.5	34.9	37.0	41.6	47.8

Source: *Social Trends*, vol. 23, 1993, p. 100

4   For all age groups and social classes *women have generally lower mortality*; although both sexes are afflicted by similar causes of death, male mortality is higher for most of these (Figures 12.1 and 12.2). However, women tend to suffer more chronic and acute illness than men, and are more likely than men to assess their own health as poor.

5   There is some evidence that the *'mortality gap'* between those at the top and bottom of the occupational classes may be increasing. This may be significant for explanations of inequalities in health.

6   Patterns of health inequalities relating to 'race' or ethnic group are less clear, partly because there has been less research and partly because findings may be complicated by birth outside the UK. Findings suggest variations in mortality rates and morbidity both between minority ethnic groups and between the latter and the 'indigenous' population.

As was suggested at the start of this chapter, these findings are compounded by geography. Additionally, they are also evident in health care. These two themes come together in the *inverse care*

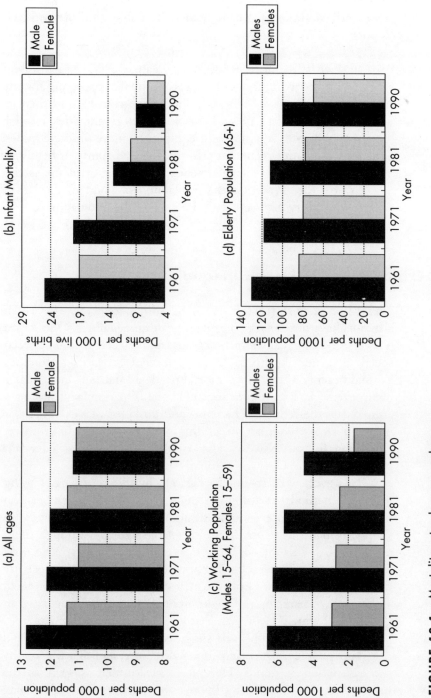

FIGURE 12.1 Mortality rates by age and sex.

Source: (for 1961, 1971, 1981) *Social Trends*, vol. 23, 1993, p. 18; (for 1990) OPCS Mortality Statistics: General DH1, no. 24, p. 6

law identified almost a decade before the publication of the Black Report:

> In areas with most sickness and death, general practitioners have more work, longer lists, less hospital support and inherit more traditions of clinically ineffective consultation than in the healthiest areas; and hospital doctors shoulder heavier caseloads with less staff and equipment, more obsolete buildings and suffer recurrent crises in the availability of beds and replacement staff. These trends can be summed up as the inverse care law: that the availability of good medical care tends to vary inversely with the need of the population served.
>
> (Tudor Hart 1971)

Explanations of health inequalities

The Black Report (DHSS 1980) identified four ways in which attempts have been made to explain health inequalities. One stance has been to dismiss any apparent 'cause and effect' relation between social class and health as a measurement *artefact* – produced by indifferent health and mortality data and an inadequate/ inconsistent classification of social classes. In particular it has been argued that the reduction of semi- and unskilled manual work has meant a steady contraction of this section of the labour force. Consequently, successive reclassifications of social class have not provided a sound basis for comparison (Illsley 1986).

However, since so much research, by different parties using different methods at different times, has found an association between 'class' (however defined) and health, it seems illogical to simply dismiss this as an aberration of the figures. Although there are problems with the data, these should rather indicate the need for better data, better classification, etc. Indeed, it has recently been argued that more precise categories of social grouping yield significantly greater mortality differentials than those calculated in the Black Report (Davey Smith *et al.* 1990).

An alternative approach suggests that health may *select* and distribute people in the occupational structure, and that this is why the association is found. Here it is health that is seen as the causative agent, distributing people to social classes, rather than vice versa. Ill health adversely affects the capacity for work, thus the healthy are more likely to be upwardly mobile in their jobs and the unhealthy are more likely to be downwardly mobile (Illsley 1955; Meadows 1961; Stern 1983). Since some causes of ill health are genetically transmitted, this *social* selection will be reinforced by *natural* selection as a predisposition to ill health or good health is transmitted over successive generations.

The problem with the selection argument is that the evidence to support it is both rather limited and questionable. The studies referred to above have been criticised on methodological grounds and this has led at least one review of the argument to conclude that health plays 'at best, a minor role in social mobility' (Blane 1985: 428).

Health is known to be affected by styles of living and patterns of behaviour. Dietary habits, child-rearing practices, drinking, smoking, exercise, etc. may all be relevant here. Might health differences between the classes simply be explained by variations in their *culture* and *behaviour*? Such an approach has a 'common sense' appeal; but may have two undesirable consequences. First, there may be a tendency to 'blame the victims' by focusing on explaining inequalities of health in terms of people's 'bad' health behaviour (eating the wrong foods; drinking or smoking too much; not taking enough exercise, etc.) and ignoring the many and varied reasons why people are often forced to behave in particular ways. Second, and consequently, policy may then become mainly directed at improving 'bad' health behaviour and ignore the real disparities in the distribution of health resources. In short, the behavioural explanation begs the question of why people may have habits that are detrimental to their health. Those on very low incomes may have far less choice about where and how they live.

This last point overlaps to some extent with the fourth type of explanation. *Material deprivation* may be associated with such factors as poor housing, diet and environment, unemployment and stress (for an overview see Blackburn (1991: 29–50)). Links between class and health could be said to exist because poverty is directly detrimental to health. This also 'makes sense'. Historically, as standards of living have improved, longevity has increased and disease has been reduced. Looking elsewhere in the world today, it is evident that the highest rates of death and disease are usually where standards of living are lowest. There is a problem here, though. If absolute poverty is *the* cause of ill health, improved standards of living should impact most clearly at the 'bottom' of the class structure, closing the health gap. Yet this does not appear to have happened.

However, if deprivation is viewed as *relative* things may become clearer. Although the lot of the poor has improved, so has that of the better off: thus, by the time Classes IV and V reach a standard previously enjoyed by Classes I and II, the latter group have 'moved on' and the gap remains. Although the health risks for Classes IV and V may change, they always remain *greater* than for those in the higher classes.

It was, then, *relative material deprivation* that the Black Report saw as the most important factor in explaining the links between social class and health: and its recommendations were couched accordingly. Thirty-seven recommendations were made

KEY TERMS

Absolute poverty and deprivation

Rest on the notion that poverty should be defined with reference to a minimum sustenance standard of living that remains fairly constant over time. Falling below this standard would place a person in absolute poverty and prolonged exposure would threaten their physical survival. They would experience absolute deprivation. It follows that absolute poverty will often have multiple dimensions (in housing, work, diet and environment).

Relative poverty and deprivation

Are based on the idea that poverty is relative to what are regarded as acceptable living standards for a society. Thus the definition of poverty changes over time; and those not able to enjoy what are currently regarded as adequate living conditions or amenities may be said to be poor. Groups may be said to be relatively deprived when compared with those who are better off.

TABLE 12.3 The Black Report – summary of recommendations

1 Need for Information and Research on:

- Child development (especially nutrition and accidents)
- Health-related behaviour (smoking, diet, exercise, alcohol consumption, etc.)
- Work-related health hazards
- Extent/nature of disabilities
- Indicators for health/social conditions
- Interaction of social factors over time and for small areas

2 Improved Planning of Health/Personal Social Services via:

Nationwide, but district-based promotion of:

- Health/welfare of mothers and children
- Care of disabled and elderly people outside institutional care
- Availability of screening services, recreational facilities in inner cities, and preventive health education programmes

Additional funding proposed for 10 locally-based health and social welfare development programmes in deprived areas

3 The Wider Strategy

(a) Comprehensive anti-poverty strategy:

- Target abolition of child poverty by 1990
- Fairer distribution of resources/wealth
- Encourage self-dependence, skill and autonomy: right to employment as a basis for these

(b) Policies for families and children:

- Raise child and maternity benefits; introduce infant care allowance
- Statutory provision for child day care
- Free nutritional school meals and milk
- Child accident prevention programme

(c) Policies in the wider community:

- A comprehensive disability allowance
- Improved health and safety at work
- More and better quality housing

(d) Co-ordination of government policy:

- Integration of health policy at Cabinet level
- Establish a government-funded, but independent Health Development Council to advise on and plan health policies

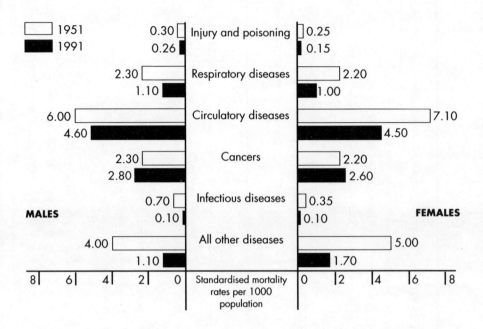

FIGURE 12.2   Selected causes of death: by sex, 1951, 1991 (UK)
Source: Social Trends, vol. 23, 1993, p. 97

(Table 12.3). These focused on three areas: the need for more information and research; improving the planning of health and personal social services, with emphasis on prevention, primary care and community health; and, third, an increase in benefits designed to radically improve the material conditions of poorer social groups, particularly children and people with disabilities.

The response

The report was submitted to the new Conservative government's Secretary of State in April 1980. The Government refused to endorse the report's recommendations due to what were seen as unrealistic costs, and the Government's judgement on the effectiveness of such expenditure. Continued concern for inequalities in health in British society, however, soon gave rise to an increasing number of studies on the subject.

The need to update the evidence led to the publication of *The Health Divide* by the Health Education Council in 1987. This report was commissioned by the Health Education Council to review the evidence on health inequalities and the progress made with the recommendations of the Black Report (DHSS 1980). The study concluded that in relation to information and research, although improvements had been made in some areas, the deficiencies had largely not been addressed. In the area of planning for health and personal social services, progress was seen to be 'painfully slow'. In relation to the wider strategy, little progress had been made in alleviating social deprivation, considered to be the underlying cause of inequalities in health.

New health challenges since the publication of the Black Report were also highlighted. High unemployment, for example, had created new health needs and social inequalities. The study also recognised the specific health needs of certain ethnic minority groups. The number of children living in poverty had also increased. All in all the report considered that 'there just has not been a recognisable national effort to tackle inequalities in health' (1988: 350).

The evidence for inequalities in health and the explanation by reference to material deprivation advocated by the Black Report and *The Health Divide* has not been supported by right-wing governments such as the Thatcher and Major administrations in the UK in the 1980s and 1990s. Rather, they have advocated the importance of individual responsibility for health behaviour. Following the White Paper *Working for Patients* (1989) and the subsequent NHS and Community Care Act (1990) their attention has focused on policies that promote the discipline of the market in health provision in an effort to increase efficiency and effectiveness in the service rather than equity. Critics such as the BMA and members of the Royal College of Surgeons have expressed concern that this may increasingly lead to greater inequalities (Whitehead 1994).

Changes to services for health promotion and ill-health prevention also carry the risk of increasing inequalities. These include increases in prescription charges, reductions in payments to dentists for NHS patients making NHS dental services increasingly difficult to access, and removal of free eye tests for the over 18s unless exempt. Even in the long-awaited health policy for England, the White Paper *The Health of the Nation* (DoH 1992), the targets for the reduction of ill health and early death in coronary heart disease and stroke, cancers, accidents, mental health and HIV and AIDS considerably downplayed evidence for a link between poverty and ill health. Rather it sought to improve the nation's health through the identification of lifestyle factors that contribute to mortality and ill health. Thus, *The Health of the Nation* sought to promote individual responsibility for health rather than acknowledge the link between economic and social deprivation and health. Adopting this behaviouralist strategy has meant a failure to address realistically the considerable health needs of large groups of the population; it has also, of course, meant that the enormous expenditure requirements such a policy would inevitably entail, particularly in an increasingly ageing society, are avoided.

Current issues and concerns

Political, economic and social trends since 1980 have often meant that reviews of inequalities in health since the Black Report have not been optimistic. Despite a 50 per cent rise in average income in the population since between 1979 and 1991 and a doubling of income amongst the wealthiest tenth of the population, more than one-fifth of the population live on less than half the national average income (Goodman and Webb 1994). This has been due to rising unemployment, a widening in the distribution of earnings, and changes to the tax-benefits system (Jenkins 1994). The cost of the health service had grown steadily from its inception but this has been exacerbated in recent years by what Black has described as 'covert denationalisation' and the financial consequences of applying an internal market (Black 1993: 1630).

see p. 37

Major social and economic changes have also, over the last decade, placed an ever increasing demand on health resources as a result of continued high levels of unemployment, a growing proportion of families experiencing poverty, more single-parent families, the continuing growth in the proportion of elderly people in the population, and the greater numbers of homeless people. These groups have higher than average health risks. It is not surprising, therefore, that the prognosis for health inequalities in the medium term is pessimistic. Not only has the mortality gap between Class V and Class I widened since the Black Report was published. A recent study has shown that during 1981–91 inequalities in mortality widened in men and women of all age categories under 75, re-emphasising the link between mortality and material conditions rather than individual behaviour (Phillimore *et al*. 1994).

Little has been said in this chapter about the health inequalities experienced by women, and even less about those faced by minority ethnic groups. Yet women and minority ethnic groups are likely to be particularly vulnerable to the trends outlined above. It is clear that much more research is needed to specifically address such matters. Equally importantly, although the Black Report identified material deprivation as the main source of health inequalities, a recent review felt obliged to still describe this area as one of research 'neglect', with too many researchers still preferring to focus on lifestyle and selection (Davey Smith *et al*. 1990).

Davey Smith *et al*. (1990) reviewed four areas where new information has become available since the publication of the Black Report: the use of alternative measures of socioeconomic position to index mortality risk; the collection of morbidity data; the comparison of inequalities in Britain with those in other industrialised countries; and greater understanding of the causes of the differentials. Their conclusions were:

1   Widening social class mortality differences.
2   Improved measurement of socioeconomic position shows greater inequalities in mortality.
3   Health inequalities are evident in all countries that collect relevant data.
4   Social selection and artefact explanations do not account for mortality differentials.
5   Class-related inequalities exist both during life and for length of life.
6   Trends in the distribution of income suggest further widening of mortality differentials may be expected.

CONCLUSION

This chapter has examined concepts of health inequality. Considerable problems remain in the measurement and study of this subject with particular controversy haunting the quest for explanations for the distribution of health and ill health. Ill health may sometimes lead to a fall in income; changes in class composition (and categorisation) complicate investigation and it is undoubtedly true that individuals may enhance their health by modifying their habits and behaviour. Yet relative material deprivation remains the most compelling explanation for health inequalities and the only one that satisfactorily addresses the persistent pattern of health inequalities in Britain today.

The ethos of government policy has not been responsive to this problem. In particular, little has been done to address the extensive inequalities in income, opportunity and resource distribution that underpin the distribution of health and ill health. Far from child poverty having been eliminated, it has grown; industrial accidents and illnesses persist; the elderly and disabled often remain severely disadvantaged; and the welfare/benefit system is not alleviating these problems to any significant degree. This prospect would seem to justify the conclusion that 'There just has not been a recognizable national effort to tackle inequalities in health' (Whitehead 1988: 350).

EXERCISES

1 Identify and discuss the limitations of the concept of social class.

2 Compare and contrast the cases for and against the four types of explanation for health inequality put forward by the Black Report.

3 Using evidence from your local area, what support can you find for the existence of an inverse care law?

4 Identify the health inequalities underlying the topics chosen for the *Health of the Nation* initiative.

Guided Reading

As a follow-up to the material in this chapter, it is essential to give a thorough reading to Townsend *et al.* (1988), the compendium publication of the *Black Report* (DHSS 1980) and *The Health Divide* (Health Education Council 1987). Blackburn (1991) is a useful overview of the relationship between poverty and health while Blaxter (1990) examines the relationship between lifestyle, behaviour and health.

Chapter 13

Economics
and health care

- Nancy North

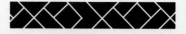

- Efficiency, effectiveness and equity

- Cost and benefit

- Quality adjusted life years

- The limitations of health economics

This chapter introduces key concepts from health economics and examines their application to the NHS.

T HOUGH GOVERNMENTS have always been concerned about efficiency in the NHS, constraints in health care spending since the mid-1970s have intensified the need to ensure that resources are put to the best possible use. After 1979 the Conservative governments emphasised the need to reduce the cost of the welfare state in relation to other items of government expenditure whilst using available resources to best effect. Their central idea was that competition would promote this goal. Consequently, as Chapter 10 has shown, the Government introduced reforms in 1990 which attempted to create a pseudo-market in health care.

This chapter will describe and evaluate concepts, taken from the discipline of health economics, which underpin the operation of today's NHS. These concepts will be considered in the context of the challenges facing purchasers and providers of health care. Though these concepts inform managerial and clinical decisions, they are not without limitations. These will be discussed at the end of the chapter.

Economic concepts

Words such as 'efficiency' and 'effectiveness' pervade the NHS. They have precise meanings in economic terms but are difficult goals to achieve. In the context of the NHS they have to be interpreted in relation to the broadest concern of the service: improving the health of the nation. Yet they also need to take account of the way in which this concern is interpretated and acted on by health care purchasers.

KEY TERMS

Efficiency

Describes a simple relationship between inputs and outputs. Ward A may be considered more efficient than ward B if, other things such as bed numbers and staff ratios being equal, ward A has a higher bed occupancy rate than ward B.

Effectiveness

Describes the relationship between outcomes and specifiable goals. If the goal of both wards is to cure patients, but more patients die on ward A than B or are discharged prematurely with complications resulting, then clearly ward B is more effective.

The task of health care providers is to become both more efficient and effective.

Efficiency

Efficiency can be separated into productive and allocative efficiency. At its simplest, productive efficiency describes the situation where, for any given input of resources, the greatest possible output is achieved. Alternatively, a service is efficient if the same output is achieved with a reduction of resources. Thus it expresses a crude relationship between inputs and outputs (e.g. bed-occupancy levels; patients seen in an out-patients' clinic), which by itself is of limited use.

Allocative efficiency relates to the distribution of resources so that patients enjoy better health as a result. It would be pointless for the NHS to endorse expenditure on a new treatment unless it could be proven that patients receive some benefit from it. As Culyer states: 'if resources are used up on ineffective care, or even on relatively ineffective care, then resources are denied to care that is effective and that must ... reduce the overall impact of health care' (Culyer 1991: 1253).

Maximum allocative efficiency would be reached where a health care purchaser could not improve the overall health of its resident population by switching resources from one programme to another. For example, if by switching funds to pay for relatively minor operations from acute surgical units to general practices, health care purchasers could increase the numbers treated for the same costs and outcomes, this would be considered to be a more efficient allocation of resources. In theory, if the same result were achieved across all programmes, maximum allocative efficiency would be realised.

Effectiveness

It should be obvious from the above discussion that the concept of efficiency has to be closely linked with that of effectiveness. Effectiveness in health care is related to the identification of improved health status as a consequence of a specific intervention, for example:

- 90 per cent of children on a GP's list achieving immunity from diphtheria, tetanus and polio as a result of the immunisation programme
- 85 per cent of patients suffering moderate stroke (as defined by diagnostic protocol) being rehabilitated to the level where they can perform specified self-care tasks
- six weeks after having toenails removed, 96 per cent of patients report full relief from symptoms and have no re-growth of the nail.

Different immunisation programmes may produce different degrees of immunity at different costs. Similarly the success rates of rehabilitation units or minor surgery may vary along with costs. Cost-effectiveness studies (see below) can reveal these differences and expose the option which gives the best results for a specified outcome, against costs. Choosing the most cost-effective treatment is important although in theory overall allocative efficiency might be increased if, by selecting a less costly programme, the resources released achieved greater benefit by being allocated elsewhere.

> **'Costs'**
>
> In economics, the term 'cost' refers to whatever is sacrificed in order to achieve or produce something. This involves the resources lost to other possible projects and includes social costs (e.g. the costs to a relative, of discharging a patient home early).
>
> Where the word 'cost' appears in this chapter, it is used to indicate a much simpler concept, for example, the expenditure necessary to provide a treatment or health care programme.

Equity

A third term, not yet mentioned, is equity. According to Culyer (1991), there are two types of equity. *Horizontal equity* exists where individuals with equal need are treated equally. For example, someone suffering from appendicitis in Bangor could expect similar treatment as someone so afflicted in Birmingham. There are difficulties in living up to this ideal. Differences in waiting-list lengths for non-urgent treatment is one example where horizontal equity is not achieved. *Vertical equity* applies where individuals with greater needs are treated relatively more favourably to compensate for the original deficit. An example of the health service striving to achieve this would be the additional funding of primary care in deprived areas; it is also evident in health promotion and health surveillance programmes which target vulnerable groups.

Clearly, the concepts of efficiency, effectiveness and equity are interwoven. In terms of producing a service which meets the general needs of the population, health care programmes must strive to meet pre-set goals (effectiveness). Those goals may contribute to the broader aim of horizontal or vertical equity in provision. However, desired outcomes should be achieved at the least possible cost; in this way resources are not squandered and can be put to use elsewhere. Stated in this matter-of-fact way, it may appear an easy process. However, although there remains a political commitment to equity within the NHS, the emphasis in much of the application of health economics has tended to be on the concepts, measurements and tools which can be used to make an organisation more efficient and effective.

The health care context

Improving efficiency and effectiveness in health care affects all levels of the service, from those who decide which services to provide, in what quantity and in which order of priority, to the clinicians at ward or directorate level, who must determine the most effective mix of resources (e.g. staff, drugs, equipment) and the uses to which they are put (e.g. treatment protocols).

Health care purchasers and GP Fundholders (GPFHs) act as agents for the local community or the patients on their practice list. Whilst health care purchasers commission services on behalf of populations and GPFHs for individuals, both have limited funds and a moral obligation to make sure that they allocate the money wisely between services or patients. It would not be advisable for a purchaser to spend all its resource allocation on coronary surgery and hip operations for its population whilst ignoring the need for such things as community services, health promotion and maternity care. Nor would a GPFH be sensible in spending allocated funds on the first hundred patients seen in the financial year, whatever the severity of their case. Essentially the problem is twofold: budgets must be spent wisely and for maximum benefit, and budgets must not be overspent.

In an ideal market, health care purchasers would be able to exercise some choice over which trusts or private health care organisations they select to provide health care services. Decisions about where contracts are placed may be based on a number of criteria:

1   How effective is the provider? Are the outcomes of specific treatments deemed to be good or, for example,
    – after a procedure, do more patients than on average die in Trust X?
    – are more patients readmitted following complications?

- does Trust Y send patients home to the care of the GP prematurely?

2   How efficient is the provider? How many patients can be treated for a specific amount of money? For the same amount of money, how many patients can nearby Trust X treat, compared with Trust Y in the next health authority?

3   How is equity of access affected? If distant Trust Y is more economic (less costly) though equally as effective in treatment outcomes as Trust X, what importance should be placed on the inconvenience to patients?

Both purchasers and providers therefore need to find out the answers to questions about efficiency and effectiveness. Purchasers need to know to make sensible purchasing decisions. Providers need to know in order to improve their market position. In order to do this the costs of services and of individual treatments will need to be established and some evaluation of their success undertaken. Comparisons may then be made with alternative forms of delivery or treatment. Health economics supplies concepts and 'tools' which may help with this complicated task.

Costs and benefits

In order to steer any organisation towards greater efficiency and effectiveness, it is important to know the costs of producing a good or in the case of the NHS, a treatment or service, and its value. In the private sector the value or utility of a product is registered by what it sells for on the market. In the case of welfare, some notional value has to be placed on the benefit derived from a health care intervention. This is a complex and essentially subjective task.

Increasingly managers will need to know not only the *total costs* of a service or series of procedures, and the *average costs* for treating a patient. They will also want to know whether costs are going up or down in each successive case treated. These are termed *marginal costs*. If the marginal costs (the costs of producing the last unit, whether it is a hip-replacement operation or day-centre place) are increasing, it may be more sensible for the trust to subcontract hip operations to another hospital where the price (cost) is lower.

TABLE 13.1   Total, average and marginal costs

Number of procedures	Total costs (£s)	Average costs (£s)	Marginal costs (£s)
1	20	20	20
2	36	18	16
3	48	16	12

Even where only average costs are known for a predicted volume of patients, it is possible to fix contracts more accurately, thereby ensuring that overfunding or underfunding of providers is avoided. The system of diagnostic related groups (DRGs) constitutes one relatively sophisticated attempt at this task. DRGs categorise patients in acute hospitals according to a number of variables including principal diagnosis, additional complications and other conditions present, surgical procedures, age, sex, and condition at discharge. The resulting groups are designed to be clinically coherent and 'iso-resource', that is they should result in a similar pattern of resource use. Of course they are not, since some patients will recover more quickly than others, but DRGs reflect average rather than individual costs.

Managers applying concepts from health economics to the NHS need to match knowledge of costs with an assessment of the benefits of particular treatments. *Cost–benefit analysis* tries to place a monetary value on the many benefits and costs of the option. For example, a cost–benefit analysis of domiciliary as opposed to residential care in the community would not simply look at the costs of keeping someone in a nursing home as opposed to providing home helps and community nurses on a daily basis. It would draw up a balance sheet which would include, amongst other things, an attempt to 'cost' the individual's preferences, the relative contribution of family, friends and neighbours, the cost of respite or day care and the support by primary health care or social services in either option.

Cost–benefit analysis enables comparisons between different options yielding different benefits, because it quantifies or costs those benefits. Those programmes or treatments that can offer the greatest benefit-to-cost ratio are accorded the highest priority. It would be inefficient to offer the service or treatment where the costs were greater than the value of the benefits received. However, whilst cost–benefit analysis might appear an attractive exercise, knowledge about health care costs and, particularly, health care benefits, is in its infancy in the NHS. In addition cost–benefit analyses are expensive exercises and are consequently impractical for much health care analysis.

Such limitations apply equally to *cost-effectiveness analysis*. Assuming that the benefits outweigh costs, cost-effectiveness analysis allows managers to compare the costs of different services or treatments for a particular condition which have broadly similar outcomes or the outcomes of different treatments for a particular condition which have similar costs. Cost-effectiveness analysis is very useful for identifying best value for money between treatments for one complaint or the most effective way of organising a programme. However, it cannot help choices between procedures for different complaints.

A third approach to the joint assessment of costs and benefits is *cost-utility analysis*. Perhaps the best known variant of this approach is the notion of the 'quality-adjusted life years' (QALYs). QALYs are a way of democratising the view of what is of value in a health care intervention. As well as identifying the cost of a procedure, they attempt to assess the benefits gained and the life span of those benefits. In placing a value on benefits, not only are the opinions of doctors sought, but those of other health care professionals and the wider population. These are incorporated within the QALY formula.

St Leger *et al.* (1992) state that the calculation of QALYs includes:

- changes in survival or life expectancy
- improvement in the quality of life (related to the degree of disability and/or distress)
- the costs of the procedure

For interventions where the purpose is not to save life, the duration of benefit from the procedure (for example, the 'life' of a knee prosthesis) rather than the patient's remaining life span, would contribute to the calculation. The quality of life, calculated from a range of opinion, is given a rating between 0 (death) to 1, then multiplied by the predicted life expectancy or years of benefit attributable to the procedure. Minus values record states where life is assumed to be worse than death (e.g. brain death but respiratory function; an unrecoverable coma). Thus, a patient expected to live 15 years in perfect health after an operation would rate 15 QALYs; someone benefiting from a procedure for 20 years with a rating of 0.25 = 5 QALYs. Following calculation of the QALY, cost is incorporated into the equation. The procedure is costed and divided by the QALY rating to find cost of producing each QALY.

TABLE 13.2   Some costs per QALY at 1983–4 prices

Intervention/procedure	Cost per QALY
Smoking cessation advice from GP	167
Hip replacement	750
GP control of hypertension	1700
Coronary artery bypass graft for moderate angina with three-vessel disease	2400
Hospital haemodialysis	14000

Source: Maynard (1987)

The limitations of health economics

Pricing health is not a simple matter. Assessing the total costs of a programme or treatment is difficult enough; having sufficiently sensitive data and the technology to identify marginal costs is more complex and carries a cost of its own. Decisions about benefits and costs accruing from a particular programme or treatment require value judgements and essentially 'value judgements made by economists are no different from value judgements made by anyone else' (Green 1990: 276). Trying to make this process more objective (as in QALYs) or democratic (see Klein 1989b) brings its own problems. Other factors which may need to be considered, such as equity and accessibility, call for finely tuned judgements about resource allocation which can be informed, but not achieved, by research studies and economic formulae.

QALYs suffer particular problems. First, there is a problem of how precisely to establish the quality of life after medical interventions. Some research surveys have been criticised for forcing respondents to answer in particular ways (Klein 1992; Fitzpatrick and Dunnell 1992). The QALY method also assumes that preferences do not change over time or in different contexts, for example, sufferers may hold a different view about the value of life following a treatment than non-sufferers. Some information about procedures, such as survival or quality of life, may not be known and different centres may produce different outcomes. It may not be accurate or ethical to apply data from groups to individual cases. Furthermore, recovery and permanent rehabilitation can be very idiosyncratic; much also might depend on the patient's overall condition before the intervention and the environment after. There are also ethical considerations. Rawles (1989) asserts that increased survival is given no greater weighting in calculations than relief of distress or disability. He criticises also the fact that QALYs value life only in terms of absence of suffering.

Economists acknowledge that the QALY system is flawed and requires further research (Maynard 1987). However, they argue that it is better to have some visible criteria for decision-making and debate rather than to blur issues or permit unchallenged medical control of society's scarce resources. Culyer (1991) contends that, regardless of methodological difficulties, some redistribution from high- to low-cost QALYs would improve allocative efficiency in the NHS.

CONCLUSION

Resources are scarce while demand for health care appears to be infinite. Given that health care should be available to all on the basis of need rather than the ability to pay, some prioritisation of provision will be required. In order to manage this effectively the various costs and benefits of providing health care need to be identified. But health economics is a far from perfect science. Neither element in the basic cost-versus-benefit equation is well understood or amenable to easy measurement. Existing data are very imperfect and the assessment of health care benefits or outcomes are contentious. Nevertheless, health economics is increasingly important in allocation decisions.

EXERCISES

1 Discuss the costs and benefits of applying the principles of health economics to the NHS.

2 Write down what problems you think may be associated with the development of QALY ratings.

Guided Reading

Gray (1993) uses a clear and accessible style to offer an alternative, more contextualised coverage of some key concepts developed in this chapter. Robinson (1993a) provides an excellent introduction to those economic concepts which can help to inform health care decisions, while Robinson (1993b), the final article in a series of six, identifies the place of health economics in today's NHS. For those interested in developing their knowledge further, articles 2 to 5 in this series (to be found in intermediate editions of the *British Medical Journal*) offer a more detailed discussion of the economic concepts outlined in Robinson's first article.

Chapter 14

Partnerships in care: the health and social care interface

■ Nancy North

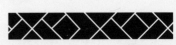

- Interagency collaboration

- Professional interaction

- The NHS reforms and collaboration

This chapter examines the development of collaboration between agencies involved in the provision of health care, with a particular emphasis on community care in the period since the 1989–90 health care reforms.

WORKING IN A HOSPITAL is a comparatively self-contained experience; the numerous professionals work in relative proximity, communication is theoretically simpler and individual roles and responsibilities are usually well understood. However, people who need care now spend shorter periods in hospital and supporting them in the community is likely to be a much more involved process, perhaps requiring the contribution of several different agencies.

The changes introduced by the NHS and Community Care Act, 1990, have made it more likely that individuals will be supported in their own homes rather than being admitted to residential care. At the same time the encouragement of a more mixed provision of welfare, with a greater role for voluntary and commercial agencies in the provision of non-institutional care, means that key workers or care managers who arrange care for vulnerable clients, will need the co-operation of several agencies.

Such collaboration operates at more than one level. It involves agencies first recognising the need for collaboration and supporting the necessary processes to ensure this. Secondly, it is also about shared understanding between different professionals and the valuing of each other's contribution to care work. This chapter will explore the past difficulties of collaboration over care, the challenging requirements of current community care policy which demand greater efforts on the part of all concerned, and some of the ways in which co-ordination of care in the community might be achieved. In doing so it will focus on two levels: co-ordination between agencies (the *strategic* level) and collaboration between workers in the NHS, personal social services and independent sector (the *operational* level).

Collaboration – the past record

Strategic collaboration

see p. 157

The importance of effective collaboration between the NHS and the personal social services was recognised in the 1974 reorganisation of the NHS. This reorganisation was partly an attempt to rationalise local authority and health service responsibilities for care provided in the community. Local authorities surrendered responsibility for certain services, among them district nursing and health visiting, but retained control of the personal social services. It was hoped that the creation of area health authorities with the same boundaries as county councils (shires), metropolitan district councils (cities) or the London boroughs, would smooth the way for what was a statutory obligation on health and local authorities to co-operate. These arrangements excluded Northern Ireland where the health and personal social services are integrated. In addition to statutory oligation, there was overlapping membership of authorities and the establishment of *joint consultative committees* to help co-ordinate community care. In 1976 the Government tried to encourage co-operation further with the introduction of *joint finance* between the NHS and personal social services for community care initiatives.

The success of these ventures was limited. Hunter and Wistow (1987) reported that although there were some notable joint projects, these were isolated and the product of collaboration at the level of practice, rather than comprehensive approaches adopted by authorities. Similarly, a joint working party of the National Association of Health Authorities (NAHA) and local authorities commented that progress had been disappointing though all concerned (health, local authorities and voluntary agencies) had recognised the need for collaboration (NAHA 1985).

In 1986 the Audit Commission was asked to report on community care. It delivered an analysis (Audit Commission 1986), which in addition to being critical of the lack of progress in community care, identified two central problems. First, responsibility for care was fragmented between different tiers within the NHS and within local authorities. This complicated negotiations with other agencies and, as a consequence, joint planning arrangements were elaborate and time-consuming. In particular, the disappearance of area health authorities in the 1982 NHS reorganisation, and with it the loss of coterminous boundaries with local authorities, had resulted in health authority representation on joint planning committees being devolved to the more numerous district health authorities.

The second problem identified by the Audit Commission was that the above difficulties were exacerbated by different priorities and styles of management within each agency. Much of the attention of health authorities was focused on acute provision whilst the personal social services (PSS) had to respond to the increasing legislation in child care. The voluntary sector variously had to address the roles of service provider and pressure group whilst the private sector needed to realise a return on investment. In addition management style and the degree of managerial autonomy between the NHS and PSS were different. Since 1983 NHS managers had had more freedom to make certain planning decisions. They were also driven by performance reviews to achieve results. The more cautious approach of local authority managers created frustrations. The contemporaneous period of financial restraint and retrenchment meant there was a reluctance to develop new and theoretically costly schemes. This in turn dampened enthusiasm for joint initiatives in care. Proceedings were characterised by: 'hard negotiations and "horse trading" between separate, self contained and often fiercely independent organisations rather than joint planning and sharing of resources between partners' (Audit Commission 1986: 60). It can be argued therefore, that the record of joint planning of community care in the mid-1980s reflected collaborative failure at the strategic level. The next section will discuss relationships between those who provide direct care and support for the client.

Operational collaboration

The picture regarding operational collaboration is complex. As the Audit Commission (1986) identified, there was evidence of dynamic co-operation at local level. McKinstry (1987), a Scottish GP, extolled the benefits of a successful ten-year liaison between his practice primary health care team and social workers. Similarly Corney (1982) also found evidence of successful working where a social worker was attached to a practice. There are, however, indications elsewhere of qualitatively different interactions. In a period covering December 1987 to May 1989 Sheppard (1992) examined contacts between social workers and GPs and community psychiatric nurses (CPNs) and GPs. He found that there were substantially more CPN/GP contact episodes than social worker/GP contact and the nature of the contact was different. CPN/GP pairs were primarily involved in passing on information about clients whilst SW/GP contacts were more likely to engage in discussions about therapeutic goals and intervention. In both contacts with SWs and CPNs the GP was unlikely to make the initial approach. Auluck and Iles (1991) found low referral rates between hospital midwives and hospital social workers. This was more pronounced for clients of Asian origin. Moreover, 50 per cent of midwifery staff held a poor opinion of social workers and the effectiveness of the service; a few described social workers as having a patronising attitude towards midwives.

In addition to empirical research findings there is evidence about breakdowns in communication between social workers and health visitors in reports of child abuse cases (Richards 1988). As a result of government concerns, a joint child abuse committee was instituted by the DHSS in 1986 as a top-level inter-agency forum for the development and supervision of child abuse policies. Case conferences of at-risk children (and adults) are held regularly between a variety of agencies, but failures still occur. The Butler-Sloss Inquiry (1988) investigated the over-zealousness of the health and social services authorities in taking excessive numbers of children into care on suspicion that they had been sexually abused. It identified a pivotal breakdown in communication and collaboration between various disciplines.

The discussion so far has focused on two levels of collaboration (strategic and operational), but there is little doubt that they are interrelated. Strategic co-ordination of services brings together various agencies and results in multi-disciplinary activity. Joint initiatives at grass-roots level can pioneer more extensive collaborative efforts. Common sense as well as research evidence suggests that shared working can break down barriers and improve collaboration.

BOX 14.1

Child abuse cases – reports of inquiry

Maria Colwell: *Report of the Committee of Inquiry into the Care and Supervision provided in relation to Maria Colwell*, London: HMSO, 1974.

Jasmine Beckford: *A Child in Trust. The Report of the Panel of Inquiry into the Circumstances surrounding the Death of Jasmine Beckford*, London: Brent Borough Council, 1985.

Kimberley Carlile : *A Child in Mind: Protection of Children in a Responsible Society. Report of the Commission of Inquiry into the Circumstances Surrounding the Death of Kimberley Carlile*, London: Greenwich Borough Council, 1987.

Tyra Henry: *Whose Child? The Report of the Panel Appointed to Inquire into the Death of Tyra Henry*, London: Lambeth Borough Council, 1989.

Effective collaboration

Effective communication and co-operation is not simply a product of 'set piece' situations, such as case conferences. It also requires that those involved appreciate the contribution that others can make. There are a number of reasons why the various professional groups working in health and community care appear unable to value each other's work fully. Perhaps the most fundamental one is that the understanding occupational groups have of the others' roles is limited and often misconceived.

Different professions have different priorities and their way of working reflects this. The DHSS Report, *Collaboration in Community Care* (1978) commented that NHS staff work relatively quickly, make decisions for their patients and provide treatment which is obvious in its effect. By contrast social workers allow their clients to determine the pace at which they work, stress non-judgemental attitudes and have less obvious means of remedial action. These might seem somewhat stereotypical views on the part of the working party, but they resonate with other explanations of conflicts between professional groups. Huntingdon (1981) suggests occupational cultures and the particular expectations they place on members create divisions, particularly between GPs and social workers.

The professionalising tendencies of both nursing and social work require that each demarcates appropriate professional territory. Dingwall (1983) refers to the professionalising strategies of exclusion and inclusion, whereby group tasks central to the character of the occupation are defended whilst attempts are made to achieve similar status with other occupations, or surpass them. This requires a celebration of a profession's efficacy which can degrade into negative stereotypical views of rival groups. Empirical support for this can be found in Auluck and Iles' study which revealed that social workers were viewed by some nurses as 'incompetent, inefficient, naive, inconsistent and too emotionally involved with clients' (Auluck and Iles 1991: 53).

Partnerships and the mixed economy of welfare

The organisational context of community care which existed in the mid-1980s has now changed dramatically. The NHS and Community Care Act, 1990, nominated local authorities as lead agencies in community care, charged with enabling and purchasing (later softened to commissioning) community care, rather than providing actual services. The voluntary agencies and private sector contract with local authority social services to provide social care. So that unnecessary duplication or gaps do not appear in provision, health and local authorities in England are required to consult and wherever possible, produce joint plans based on joint assessment. In Wales this is mandatory.

A critical element in these deliberations is deciding what constitutes health or social care. Commissioning health authorities, particularly as contracts move to cost and volume arrangements (where payment is based on a specific number of cases treated), will need to strike a balance between generosity of definition and the servicing of priority health care needs. Their decisions should be clear and well publicised. The Audit Commission's 1992 report, *The Community Revolution*, cautioned that care should be taken that agreements are acknowledged and that working practices accord with them. However, the benefits of closer association between local authority social services and health commissioners may come to more than the clarification of responsibilities. Joint commissioning of community care projects may signal success for the new arrangements for community care where joint planning singularly failed. There is mixed evidence about the degree to which this is happening. Wistow *et al.*'s (1993) survey of community care plans indicated wide variations in the degree of consultation between LAs and health authorities, with such consultation as there was often being at a draft stage.

KEY TERMS

Health care
Generally equated with actions designed to cure sickness or manage the symptoms of ill health or disability.

Social care
Relates to the non-medical interventions focused on ensuring that a person is able to lead a full social life.

The two are clearly interlinked.

At the operational level the *care manager* – an individual responsible for co-ordinating the care programmes of clients with complex needs – will play a key role in co-ordinating care from a 'menu' of providers in the voluntary/commercial sector, as well as soliciting help from primary health care team members and other community nursing services. Given some of the professional sensitivities outlined in an earlier section, which tend to encourage a defensive approach, this will require some diplomatic skill.

Both local authorities and DHAs are required to ensure stategic co-operation over multi-disciplinary assessment procedures. In the case of health care providers, requirements are to be specified in contracts. Clearly, this is advantageous to clients already living in the community, but it is essential for those patients about to be discharged from hospital into the care of social services and onto the social care budget. In making local authorities the lead agency in community care, the NHS and Community Care Act, 1990, also made them financially accountable. Thus the costs of care for patients discharged from hospital and requiring either institutional or domiciliary care, over and above what can be contributed by the patients themselves, are met from the social care budget. Concerns have been voiced that if this is inadequate in any way, social workers will be reluctant to agree to discharges and bed-blocking will result (Lelliot *et al.* 1993).

Co-operation between social services and voluntary sector providers is also secured through the contracting process, a change in culture which not all voluntary agencies relish. Whilst some welcome contractual arrangements which assure funds for a specified period, others are concerned that contracting will change the relationship many of them enjoyed with the social services departments and reduce their autonomy. Much will depend on the style adopted by the local authorities (Harding 1990), though uncertainties about the maturity of welfare markets would make aggressive contracting unadvisable. Local authorities may need to nurture whatever suitable providers they have in their patch, rather than drive them into a corner. Added to this, Wistow *et al.* (1992) found that many local authorities were themselves uncomfortable with the concept of purchasing community care.

The relationship between local authority social services departments and health providers, notably community trusts, may become contractual if trusts bid to provide services in the grey area between health and social care. An example of this is where a community trust tenders for a contract to provide a 'sitting service' for vulnerable clients whilst relatives take time off. If 'contractual webs' develop between community trusts and local authority social services departments they may provide the latter with some leverage in other forms of collaboration such as non-contractual liaison over strategic community care planning.

The health care services which trusts develop as a part of the effort to become more efficient may have important consequences for local authorities as commissioners of social care. Innovatory new developments, such as hospital-at-home services, designed to care for patients who are discharged early after in-patient treatment or who are cared for at home for longer than normal between treatment episodes, will inevitably increase demands for social care and require the attention of care managers. At a strategic level, health care providers and purchasers will need to discuss with local authorities the implications of this type of service and secure their agreement.

More generally, relationships between trusts and social services departments will be forged by the need to work together to manage a system of community care which is substantially more fragmented than before. Moreover, the projected increase in numbers of older people requiring health and social care, and the possible reduction in scale of large acute care hospitals, will increase the need for contact between staff and effective organisation. As always, success will depend on goodwill and a clear understanding of respective commitments.

In some PSS departments the job of care manager is being piloted within GP fundholding practices (Hunter 1991b). This is a sensible location given the need to communicate about clients and cultivate the benevolence of primary health care staff. GP/care manager practices also form a 'one stop shop' for clients and, as more practices computerise records, could provide excellent information about individual and neighbourhood needs if the difficulties about confidentiality and access are overcome. Hunter suggests the encouragement of GP/care manager practices may be indicative of government interest in the possibility of GP fundholding playing a more central role in community care. Since April 1993 GP fund holders have been able to purchase community nursing services; and at the end of 1994 the government announced an initiative to extend the purchasing of community services through GP fund holders. Such a concentration of decentralised purchasing may prove to be an irresistible marriage of managerial convenience and ideological aspiration.

The changes in the structure of community care outlined above will inevitably complicate communication and relationships between the professions. Sensible systems of communication between a multiplicity of providers will need to be established. There may be tensions between organisational commitments and professional loyalties. As mentioned above, one of the concerns of any profession is to maintain status and 'territory'. The necessary clarification of functions in community care may lead to defensiveness on the part of those who feel they have something to lose.

More positively, there are indications of collaborative efforts on the part of health and social services staff and the voluntary sector (King 1993). Closer contact, hopefully a routine outcome of the community care reforms, will in turn help to break down professional barriers thus producing more effective partnerships in the future.

CONCLUSION

The past difficulties of communication and collaboration in community care are well documented. They relate not only to problems at the strategic, inter-agency level, but also to difficulties experienced by those directly caring for the client. The different dimensions of the problem invoke different explanations – incompatible structures, clashes of organisational style and funding uncertainties created obstacles to the strategic planning of community care in the past. Also relevant were the different priorities of the services and the differing professional cultures of those who worked in them. The sociology of professions (Chapter 8) has much to offer the analysis.

The health service and community care reforms have fractured previous organisational structures and demanded a change in managerial styles. Professional values may become subordinated to new managerial agendas calling for different priorities and changing professional practice. Services in health and social care will be more rigorously defined and co-operation in identifying and providing for gaps in care will be essential, along with the need to ensure co-ordinated provision. The changes may bring different professional groups into contact more frequently, contributing to a breakdown of stereotypical attitudes and defensiveness. Alternatively, times of organisational change bring uncertainty and heightened sensitivity, provoking reactionary professional posturing. Future relationships in community care will depend upon present management having the necessary wisdom and skills to lay sturdy foundations.

- Evaluate this statement by the Audit Commission:

  The NHS, in its various parts, has different priorities from social services; including sometimes adopting a 'medical' rather than a 'social' model of care, focusing on short-term acute intervention rather than long-term support, and a short rather than a long time scale.

  (Audit Commission 1992: 49)

- Which 'parts' of the NHS does this analysis least describe?

- What contribution should the NHS make to community care?

Guided Reading

The Audit Commission (1992: Ch.4) maps out the agenda for collaboration today, while Allen (1991) pre-dates the changes ushered in by the Act, but gives an idea of the challenges facing authorities involved in community care. Harding (1990) comments on the changed circumstances of voluntary agencies, and Means and Smith (1994) offer a useful insight into the collaborative workings of the various agencies involved in community care.

Chapter 15

Conclusion

- Rosemary Gillespie
- Graham Moon

T HE CONTRIBUTORS TO THIS BOOK have attempted to show the ways in which health, illness and disease, far from being objective, scientific certainties, are inextricably embedded in the history, culture and social structure of human societies. The perspectives presented have been intended to provide health professionals with an introduction to health, illness and disease in a social context. We have also introduced some of the social, political and ideological debates that underpin the provision of health care in a changing society. This, it is hoped, will enable the reader to understand more fully some of the complex issues that impinge on health and the delivery of health care. It will also, it is hoped, help them to make sense of the radical changes that health care in Britain is currently undergoing following the reforms introduced in the NHS and Community Care Act, 1990.

The first section of the text brought together the social, historical, geographical and demographical issues within which health and illness are experienced, disease is diagnosed, and health care services are delivered. This highlighted the important and growing

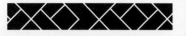

link between medicine and social science. Two models for under-standing historical changes in the prevalence of disease and the structure of the population were identified, the demographic and the epidemiological transitions. These transitions underlie the basic characteristics of the populations requiring health care in Britain today. On the one hand they relate to the reduction in infant mortality and infectious disease, whilst on the other they link to the increasing importance of cancers, heart disease and other degenerative diseases. The low birth rate and low death rate have also brought about our increasingly ageing population.

Demographic and epidemiological changes have a significant impact on the provision of care, both formal and informal. This impact is exacerbated by changing conceptions of the family. This profoundly sociological construct has undergone considerable change in the past few decades, casting doubt on the dominance of traditional notions of family and its ability to support its members during periods of illness. Today greater numbers of people live in single-parent, reconstituted or other non-traditional family structures. In addition, the role of women has undergone signifi-cant changes during the last century, although perhaps not as much as some women would like and more for some women than others. Women still remain the primary care givers in both professional and informal settings but women's 'natural' caring role within the family has increasingly been questioned.

Similar and no less far-reaching changes have affected the equally contested notion of community. The idea that communities will naturally be able to shoulder the care of sick people denies the many changes which have happened in Britain's rural and urban neighbourhoods. Taken together, the themes discussed in Chapters 1 and 2 raise a serious challenge for health care providers of the new century: who will be the care givers in the future?

The social sciences give prime consideration to the social, cultural, political and economic factors that affect health and ill-ness. In Chapter 3 we showed how changing views about health care can be interpreted using social science tools and analysis to make sense of complex issues. We showed that the rise to power of the medical model of care was a lengthy process in which a number of stages could be identified. These different stages saw the increasing importance of the medical practitioner and the progressive marginalisation of other professions and patients; they created an approach to health care which we characterised as the medical model.

We then explored critiques of the medical model before contrasting it with the broader social model of health in which health is seen in the context of wider social experience, such as poverty, homelessness, culture and the environment. We highlighted how the critics of biomedicine sought to demonstrate the ways in which medicine is not always as objective, rational and altruistic, as is often assumed. Claims about its success are not always wholly founded on sound evidence, either in an historical sense or in an economic sense. Nor is its progress unrelated to ethical issues or the concerns of capital and patriarchy. Frequently it can be seen to act in the interests of powerful professional groups such as doctors, nurses and, more recently, managers. We concluded the first part of the book by examining two sociological concepts – the sick role and stigma – which reveal the social nature of sickness.

The second section of the text provided an analysis of the ways in which individuals and groups respond to the experience of health, illness, disease and disability. Understanding illness as a social phenomenon helps explain the ways in which people come to seek help for their health problems from a variety of agencies, some of which might include the primary or secondary health care services, but may also include a range of alternative or complementary therapies or self treatments. We explored some of the complex ways in which individuals come to understand health, illness and disease and investigated the sociological factors that underpin people's behaviour when they are ill and when they seek care. Attention was drawn to the failure of much ill health to come to the attention of the primary health care services. It was suggested that this 'illness iceberg' indicated that many individuals appear to 'accommodate' their problems whilst others may seek alternative ways of treating illness that represent competing rather than subordinate belief systems which lie outside the remit of the health services.

Interaction between health professionals and patients/clients is an important area for sociological research. It has major implications for increasing our understanding of the dynamics of health care and significant potential applications in the area of promoting better care. Traditional paternalistic relationships, especially those between doctor and patient that position patients as passive and doctors as experts whose advice is unquestioningly adhered to, are increasingly being challenged. More and more patients see health professionals as sources of advice and expertise and expect greater participation in decision making. Information about clinical decisions and advice about care options are expected and an integral part of the patient taking responsibility for their own care and treatment. The interaction that takes place between health professional and patient or client can also have a significant impact on the outcome of care. This is increasingly evident as patients become more aware of their rights, in what is becoming a more consumerist, market-oriented, health-provider environment, where mutual participation may increasingly become a feature of health service provision.

Such awareness was often absent in the past. Chapter 8 examined the sociological debates surrounding the concept of the institution. Drawing mainly from the mental health literature, it was shown that routinised and ritualised care giving, such as was common in many hospitals until recently and undoubtedly still exists, was counterproductive, challenging the autonomy and rights of patients/clients. Professionalisation strategies were also subjected to critical evaluation. Professional gatekeeping and professional stereotypes were shown to have both positive and negative results as regards care giving.

The third part of the book considered the social, economic and political implications of current health policies in the UK. The 1990s constitute a time of great uncertainty and change in the health services; familiar patterns of service provision are changing and the health professional faces a bewildering array of new and sometimes job-threatening developments. Despite over forty years of the NHS, inequalities in health in British society have been shown to persist. Despite regular reforms they even appear to be increasing; it is doubtful whether recent policy developments will reverse this trend. Despite continuing increases in expenditure, the health chances for those in the lower social classes remain much worse than those in the higher social groups. Unemployment also constitutes a considerable additional health challenge.

Responsibility for health, whether individual or social, remains an area of intense political controversy. The Conservative government in Britain in the early 1990s, keen to keep welfare costs to a minimum, has sought to promote individual responsibility for health. The clear focus of policy has been on attempts to alter health-related behaviour with the White Paper *The Health of the Nation* exemplifying current thinking. Sociologists of health and health policy analysts, however, have argued that health behaviour cannot be understood in isolation. Real understanding needs to take into account the contexts in which behaviours take place; these are likely to reflect major divisions in society, such as gender, class and race, the income of a person and the type of area in which they live. Promoting individual responsibility for health behaviour without tackling the socioeconomic circumstances of people's lives constitutes victim blaming and does not provide an adequate solution to the problem of health inequalities.

In Britain health care reforms have led to considerable change in the ways in which health care services are planned, funded and delivered. Major changes in NHS management in the 1980s have been aimed at providing a more cost-effective, efficient, dynamic, responsive health service through the introduction of business practices, such as the internal market, GP fundholding and greater use of the private sector. We have seen that, although governments have always been concerned about efficiency and economy in the NHS, constraints on health care spending since the mid-1970s have intensified with an imperative to ensure that resources are used effectively and efficiently. Since 1979 the Conservative government has increasingly emphasised a need to reduce the relative cost of welfare spending as a whole, whilst using what resources are available to best effect. In the NHS this has had a significant impact leading to increased control on the service from central government, as well as on professional groups, such as doctors, nurses and other health professionals.

The changes introduced following the NHS and Community Care Act, 1990, have also had a significant impact on services to patients. People who need care now spend shorter periods in hospital and increasingly are supported in their own homes and in the community, rather than being admitted to residential long-term care. Community care often requires the contribution of several different agencies and has implications which are far reaching, particularly for women, who have historically been the prime care givers in the family and community, but increasingly are demanding equal opportunities in the workplace and society as a whole.

If there is one enduring theme which links all the contributions to this text, it is the tension between the individual and society. Social science, as distinct from behavioural science, tends to stress the role of society. In the context of health, disease and health care, this entails a recognition that much of what is taken for granted as unchallengeable or straightforward is profoundly influenced by the social context in which it is found, produced and constructed. This applies to health and to health care, to the behaviour of the sick person and the health professional, and to health policy. Context is central; by understanding it and its influence we can begin to understand the nature of health problems and the potential of different solutions to them.

Health professionals face significant challenges, at a time of intense change, tight budgetary control, performance indicators and new health challenges. They will need knowledge and skill if they are to continue to provide a high quality service in a new streamlined, increasingly business-oriented health care arena. Only through a solid understanding of the ideological, social and political issues involved can health care professionals adequately fulfil their role as both the providers of services and patient advocates, in an increasingly challenging arena.

References

Abberley, P. (1993) 'Disabled people and "normality"', in J. Swain, V. Finkelstein, S. French and M. Oliver (eds) *Disabling Barriers – Enabling Environments*, London: Open University/Sage.

Abbott, P. and Wallace, C. (1990) *Introduction to Sociology: Feminist Perspectives*, London: Routledge.

Abel-Smith, B. (1964) *The Hospitals 1800–1948*, London: Heinemann.

Abel-Smith, B. (1976) *Value for Money in Health Services*, London: Heinemann.

Abel-Smith, B. (1990) 'The first forty years', in J. Carrier and I. Kendall (eds) *Socialism and the NHS*, Aldershot: Gower.

Alderson, M. (1983) *An Introduction to Epidemiology*, London: Macmillan.

Allan, G. (1987) 'Informal networks of care', *British Journal of Social Work* 13: 417–33.

Allen, I. (1991) *Health and Social Services: The New Relationship*, London: Policy Studies Institute.

Allsop, J. (1984) *Health Policy and the National Health Service*, London: Longman.

Audit Commission (1986) *Making a Reality of Community Care*, London: HMSO.

Audit Commission (1992) *The Community Revolution: Personal Social Services and Community Care*, London: HMSO.

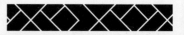

Auluck, R. and Iles, P. (1991) 'The referral process: a study of working relationships between antenatal clinic nursing staff and hospital social workers and their impact on Asian women', *British Journal of Social Work* 21: 41–61.

Baxter, J. (1994) 'Is husband's class enough? class location and class identity in the United States, Sweden, Norway, and Australia', *American Sociological Review* 59: 220–35.

Becker, M.H., Haefneer, D.P., Kasl, S.V., Kirrscht, J., Maiman, I. and Rosenstock, I.M. (1977) 'Selected psychological models and correlates of individual health related behaviours', *Medical Care* 15, 5, Supplement: 27–46.

Berger, B. and Berger, P. (1983) *The War Over the Family*, London: Hutchinson.

Berliner, H. (1985) *A System of Scientific Medicine*, New York: Tavistock.

Beveridge Report (1942) *Social Insurance and Allied Services*, Cmd. 6404, London: HMSO.

Black, D. (1993) 'The political and the personal', *British Medical Journal* 307: 1630–1.

Black, N., Boswell, D., Gray, A., Murphy, S. and Popay, J. (eds) (1987) *Health and Disease: A Reader*, London: Open University Press.

Blackburn, C. (1991) *Poverty and Health*, London: Open University Press.

Blane, D. (1985) 'An assessment of the Black Report's explanations of health inequalities', *Sociology of Health and Illness* 7, 3: 423–45.

Blaxter, M. (1984) 'Equity and consultation rates in general practice', *British Medical Journal* 6345: 1963–6.

Blaxter, M. (1990) *Health and Lifestyles*, London: Routledge.

Brand, J. (1965) *Doctors and the State*, Baltimore: Johns Hopkins Press.

Brown, G.W., Birley, J. and Wing, A. (1972) 'The influence of family life on the course of schizophrenic disorders: a replication', *British Journal of Psychiatry* 121: 241–58.

Bucquet, D., Jarman, B. and White, P. (1985) 'Factors associated with home visiting in an inner London general practice', *British Medical Journal* 290: 1480–3.

Busfield, J. (1986) *Managing Madness*, London: Hutchinson.

Butler, J. (1992) *Patients, Policies and Politics*, Milton Keynes: Open University Press.

Butler-Sloss Inquiry (1988) *Report of the Inquiry into Child Sexual Abuse in Cleveland*, Cm 412, London: HMSO.

Byrne, P.S. and Long, B.L. (1976) *Doctors Talking to Patients*, London: HMSO.

Calder, A. (1969) *The People's War*, London: Granada.

Carrier, J. and Kendall, I. (1986) 'NHS management and the "Griffiths Report"', in M. Brenton and C. Ungerson (eds) *The Year Book of Social Policy in Britain, 1985–6*, London: Routledge & Kegan Paul.

Carrier, J. and Kendall, I. (eds) (1990) *Socialism and the NHS*, Aldershot: Avebury.

Cartwright, A. and O'Brien, M. (1976) 'Social class variation in health care', in M. Stacey (ed.) *The Sociology of the NHS*, Sociological Review Monograph 22, Keele: University of Keele.

Charlton, J., Hartley, R., Silver, R. and Holland, W. (1983) 'Geographical variations in mortality from conditions amenable to medical intervention in England and Wales', *Lancet*: 1: 691–6.

Chen, L., Kleinman, A. and Ware, A. (eds) (1992) *The Health Transition*, Cambridge, MA: Harvard University Press.

Chrisman, N.J. (1977) 'The health seeking process: an approach to the natural history of illness', *Culture, Medicine and Psychiatry* 1: 351–77.

Cochrane, A.L. (1972) *Effectiveness and Efficiency*, London: Nuffield Provincial Hospitals Trust.

Cohen, S. and Scull, A. (eds) (1983) *Social Control and the State*, Oxford: Blackwell.

Conrad, P. and Schneider, J. (1980) *Deviance and Medicalisation*, St Louis: Mosby.

Corney, R.H. (1982) 'Chapter 3', in A.W. Clare and R.H. Corney (eds) *Social Work and Primary Health Care*, London: Associated Publishing.

Culyer, A.J. (1991) 'The promise of a reformed NHS: an economist's angle', *British Medical Journal* 302: 1253–6.

Davey Smith, G., Bartley, M. and Blane, D. (1990) 'The Black report on socioeconomic inequalities in health 10 years on', *British Medical Journal* 301: 373–7.

Department of Health (1989) *Working for Patients* (Cmd. 555), London: HMSO.

Department of Health (1992) *The Health of the Nation*, London: HMSO.

Department of Health and Social Security (1976) *Priorities for Health and Personal Social Services in England : a Consultative Document*, London: HMSO.

Department of Health and Social Security (1978) *Collaboration in Community Care – a Discussion Document*, Chairperson, A. Winner, London: HMSO.

Department of Health and Social Security (1979) *Patients First*, London: HMSO.

Department of Health and Social Security (1980) *Inequalities in Health: Report of a Research Working Group*, London: Department of Health and Social Security (The Black Report).

Department of Health and Social Security (1981) *Growing Older* (Cmd. 8173), London: HMSO.

Department of Health and Social Security (1983) *NHS Management Inquiry*, London: DHSS (The Griffiths Report).

Department of Health and Social Security (1987) *Promoting Better Health – the Government's Programme for Improving Primary Health Care*

(Cmd. 249), London: HMSO.

Department of Health and Social Security (1989) *Caring for People: Community Care in the Next Decade and Beyond* (Cmd. 849), London: HMSO.

Dingwall, R. (1983) 'Introduction', in R. Dingwall and P. Lewis (eds) *The Sociology of the Professions: Lawyers, Doctors and Others*, London: Macmillan.

Dingwall, R., Rafferty, A-M. and Webster, C. (1988) *An Introduction to the Social History of Nursing*, London: Routledge.

Doyal, L. (1979) *The Political Economy of Health*, London: Pluto.

Dubos, R. (1960) *Mirage of Health*, London: Allen & Unwin.

Dunnell, K. and Cartwright, A. (1972) *Medicine Takers, Prescribers and Hoarders*, London: Routledge & Kegan Paul.

Earthrowl, B. and Stacey, M. (1977) 'Social class and children in hospital', *Social Science and Medicine* 11: 83–8.

Ehrenreich, B. and English, D. (1976) *Witches, Midwives and Nurses*, London: Writers and Publishers Press.

Fitzpatrick, R. and Dunnell, K. (1992) 'Measuring outcomes in health care', in E. Beck, S. Lonsdale, S. Newman and D. Patterson (eds) *The Best of Health?* London: Chapman & Hall.

Flynn, R. (1991) 'Coping with cutbacks and managing retrenchment in health', *Journal of Social Policy* 20, 2: 215–36.

Foster, P. (1989) 'Improving the doctor/patient relationship: a feminist perspective', *Journal of Social Policy* 18, 3: 337–61.

Foucault, M. (1967) *Madness and Civilisation*, London: Tavistock.

Foucault, M. (1973) *The Birth of the Clinic*, London: Tavistock.

Freidson, E. (1970a) *Professional Dominance*, Chicago: Aldine, pp. 134–5.

Freidson, E. (1970b) *The Profession of Medicine*, New York: Dodd, Mead & Co.

Freidson, E. (1986) *Professional Powers: a Study of the Institutionalisation of Formal Knowledge*, Chicago: University of Chicago Press.

Frenk, J., Bobadilla, J., Sepulveda, J. and Cervantes, M. (1989) 'Health transition in middle income countries', *Health Policy and Planning* 4: 29–39.

Giddens, A. (1989) *Sociology*, London: Polity Press.

Gilbert, B. (1966) *Evolution of National Insurance in Great Britain*, London: Michael Joseph.

Goffman, E. (1961) *Asylums: Essays on the Social Situation of Mental Patients and Other Inmates*, New York: Anchor Books, Doubleday & Co.

Goffman, E. (1963) *Notes on the Management of Spoiled Identity*, Boston: Prentice-Hall.

Goffman, E. (1991) *Asylums*, Penguin: London.

Goodman, A. and Webb, S. (1994) *For Richer, For Poorer*, Swansea: Institute of Fiscal Studies.

Gray, A. (1993) 'Rationing and choice', in B. Davey and J. Popay (eds)

Dilemmas in Health Care, Milton Keynes: Open University Press.

Green, A. (1990) 'Health economics: are we being realistic about its value?' *Health Policy and Planning* 5: 274–9.

Griffiths, R. (1983) *NHS Management Enquiry*, London: HMSO.

Ham, C.J. (1990) *Health Policy in Britain* (3rd edition), Basingstoke: Macmillan.

Hannay, D. (1980) 'The iceberg of illness and trivial consultations', *Journal, Royal College of General Practitioners* 30: 551–4.

Haralambos, M. (1985) *Sociology: Themes and Perspectives*, London: Bell & Hyman.

Harding, T. (1990) 'A change of identity', *Insight*, 28 March, 18–20.

Harrison, S. (1988) *Managing the National Health Service: Shifting the Frontier?* London: Chapman & Hall.

Health Education Council (1987) *The Health Divide*, London: Health Education Council.

Her Majesty's Stationery Office (1993) *Social Trends*, London: HMSO.

Herzlich, C. (1973) *Health and Illness*, London: Academic Press.

Hockey, J. (1993) 'Women and health', in D. Richardson and V. Robson (eds) *Introducing Women's Studies*, London: Macmillan.

Honigsbaum, F. (1989) *Health, Happiness and Security – The Creation of the National Health Service*, London: Routledge.

Hood, C. (1991) 'A public management for all seasons?' *Public Administration* 69: 3–19.

Hugman, R. (1991a) *Power in Caring Professions*, Basingstoke: Macmillan.

Hunter, D. (1991) 'Managing medicine: a response to the "crisis"', *Social Science and Medicine* 32, 4: 441–9.

Hunter, D. (1991b) 'A policy for care – or for chaos?' *Health Service Journal*, 4 July, 101: 30–1.

Hunter, D. and Wistow, G. (1987) 'The paradox of policy diversity in a unitary state: community care in Britain', *Public Administration* Spring, 65: 3–24.

Huntingdon, J. (1981) *Social Work and General Medical Practice: Collaboration or Conflict*, London: George Allen & Unwin.

Illich, I. (1976) *Limits to Medicine*, London: Calder & Boyars.

Illsley, R. (1955) 'Social class selection and class differences in relation to stillbirths and infant deaths', *British Medical Journal* 2: 1520.

Illsley, R. (1986) 'Occupational class, selection and the production of inequalities in health', *Quarterly Journal of Social Affairs* 2, 2: 151–65.

Jenkins, S. (1994) *Winners and Losers*, Swansea: Institute of Fiscal Studies.

Jewson, N. (1976) 'The disappearance of the sick man from medical cosmology', *Sociology* 10: 225–44.

Jones, K. (1972) *A History of the Mental Health Services*, London: Routledge.

Jones, K. (1991) *The Making of Social Policy in Britain*, London: Athlone.

Jones, K. and Fowles, A. J. (1984) *Ideas on Institutions*, London: Routledge

& Kegan Paul.

Jones, K. and Moon, G. (1987) *Health, Disease and Society*, London: Routledge & Kegan Paul.

Jones, K. and Moon, G. (1992) 'Medical geography: global perspectives', *Progress in Human Geography* 16: 563–72.

Kendall, I. and Moon, G. (1990) 'Health policy', in S.P. Savage, and L. Robins (eds) *Public Policy under Thatcher*, Basingstoke: Macmillan.

Kendall, I. and Moon, G. (1994) 'Health policy and the Conservatives', in S.P. Savage, R. Atkinson and L. Robins (eds) *Public Policy in Britain*, London: Macmillan, pp. 162–81.

King, J. (1993) 'Round up 93: Implementation 5', *Community Care*, 4 February, 952: 18–19.

Klein, R. (1983) *The Politics of the National Health Service* (1st edition), London: Longman.

Klein, R. (1989a) *The Politics of the National Health Service* (2nd edition), London: Longman.

Klein, R. (1989b) 'The role of health economics', *British Medical Journal* 299: 275–6.

Klein, R. (1992) 'Warning signs from Oregon', *British Medical Journal* 304: 1457–8.

Kleinman, A. (1980) *Patients and Healers in the Context of Culture*, Los Angeles: University of California Press.

Kleinman, A. (1985) 'Indigenous systems of healing: questions for professional, popular and folk care', in J. Salmon (ed.) *Alternative Medicines: Popular and Policy Perspectives*, London: Tavistock.

Laing, R.D. (1971) *Politics and the Family*, London: Macmillan.

Leathard, A. (1990) *Health Care Provision: Past, Present and Future*, London: Chapman & Hall.

Lelliot, P., Sims, A. and Wing, J. (1993) 'Who pays for community care? The same old question', *British Medical Journal*, 16 October, 307: 991–4.

Lindow, V. (1993) 'A service user's view', in H. Wright and M. Giddey (eds), *Mental Health Nursing: From First Principles to Professional Practice*, London: Chapman & Hall.

McInstry, B. (1987) 'Successful liaison between the health team and social workers in Blackburn, West Lothian', *British Medical Journal*, 24 January, 294: 221–4.

McKeown, T. (1979) *The Role of Medicine*, Oxford: Blackwell.

McKeown, T. (1988) *The Origins of Human Disease*, Oxford: Blackwell.

McKinlay, J. (1973) 'Social networks, lay consultation and help seeking behaviour', *Social Forces* 53: 255–92.

Martin, J.P. (1984) *Hospitals in Trouble*, Oxford: Blackwell.

Maynard, A. (1987) 'Markets and health care', in A. Williams (ed.) *Health and Economics*, London: Macmillan.

Meade, M., Florin, J. and Gesler, W. (1988) *Medical Geography*, New York:

Guilford.

Meadows, S.H. (1961) 'Social class migration and chronic bronchitis', *British Journal of Social Medicine* 15: 171.

Means, R. and Smith, R. (1994) *Community Care, Policy and Practice*, London: Macmillan.

Mechanic, D. (1968) *Medical Sociology*, London: Free Press.

Mechanic, D. (1992) 'Health and illness behaviour and patient–practitioner relationships', *Social Science and Medicine* 34, 12: 1345–50.

Midelfort, E. (1980) 'Madness and civilisation in Early Modern Europe: a reappraisal of Michel Foucault', in B. Malament (ed.) *After the Reformation: Essays in Honour of J.H. Hexter*, Philadelphia: University of Pennsylvania Press.

Ministry of Health (1962) *National Health Service: A Hospital Plan for England and Wales* (Cmnd. 1604), London: HMSO.

Ministry of Health (1963) *Plans for Health and Welfare Services of the Local Authorities in England and Wales* (Cmnd. 1973), London: HMSO.

Ministry of Health (1966) *Report of the Committee on Senior Nursing Staff Structure*, London: HMSO (The Salmon Report).

Morgan, M. (1991) 'The doctor–patient relationship', in G. Scambler (ed.) *Sociology as Applied to Medicine*, London: Baillière Tindall.

Morgan, M., Calnan, M. and Manning, N. (1985) *Sociological Approaches to Health and Illness*, London: Routledge & Kegan Paul.

National Association of Health Authorities (1985) *Progress in Partnership*, London: NAHA.

National Federation of Women's Institutes (1993) *Caring for Rural Carers*, London: NFWI.

Navarro, V. (1976) *Medicine Under Capitalism*, New York: Prodist.

Nissel, M. (1987) *People Count*, London: HMSO.

Oakley, A. (1980) *Women Confined*, London: Martin Robertson.

Oakley, A. (1993) *Essays on Women, Medicine and Health*, Edinburgh: Edinburgh University Press.

Office of Population Censuses and Surveys (1993) *General Household Survey*, London: HMSO.

Omran, A. (1971) 'The epidemiological transition: a theory of the epidemiology of population change', *Millbank Memorial Fund Quarterly*, 49: 509–38.

Open University (1985a) *The Health of Nations*, London: Open University Press.

Open University (1985b) *Medical Knowledge: Doubt and Certainty*, London: Open University Press.

Open University (1993) *World Health and Disease*, London: Open University Press.

Parsons, T. (1951) *The Social System*, New York: Free Press.

Pendleton, D.A. and Bochner, S. (1980) 'The communication of medical information in general practice consultations as a function of patients' social class', *Social Science and Medicine* 14: 669–73.

Phillimore, P., Beattie, A. and Townsend, P. (1994) 'Widening inequality of health in Northern England, 1981–91', *British Medical Journal* 308: 1125–8

Pinker, R. (1966) *English Hospital Statistics 1861–1938*, London: Heinemann.

Pollitt, C., Harrison, S., Hunter, D.J. and Marnoch, G. (1991) 'General management in the NHS: the initial impact 1983–88', *Public Administration* 69: 61–83.

Ranade, W. (1994) *A Future for the NHS? Health Care in the 1990s*, London: Longman.

Rawles, J. (1989) 'Castigating QALYs', *Journal of Medical Ethics* 15: 143–7.

Renn, M. (1987) 'One step forward', *Nursing Times* 83 (24): 30–1.

Richards, M. (1988) *Key Issues in Child Abuse: Some Lessons from Cleveland and Other Inquiries*, London: National Institute of Social Work.

Robinson, R. (1993a) 'Economic evaluation and health care: what does it mean?', *British Medical Journal* 307: 670–3.

Robinson, R. (1993b) 'Economic evaluation and health care: the policy context', *British Medical Journal* 307: 994–6.

Rose, S., Kamin, L. and Lewontin, R. (1984) *Not in Our Genes*, London: Penguin.

Rosenstock, I. (1966) 'Why people use health services', *Millbank Memorial Fund Quarterly* 44: 54–127.

Rothman, D.J. (1983) 'Social control: the uses and abuses of the concept in the history of incarceration', in S. Cohen and A. Scull (eds) *Social Control and the State*, Oxford: Blackwell.

Rowden, R. (1990) 'Colouring attitudes', *Nursing Times* 86 (24): 47–8.

Royal Commission on the NHS (1979) *Report* (Cmnd. 7615), London: HMSO (Merrison Report).

Sainsbury, P. and Grad de Alarcon (1974) 'The last of community care and the burden on the family of treating the mentally ill at home', in D. Lees and S. Shaw (eds) *Impairment, Disability and Handicap*, London: Heinemann.

Savage, S.P. and Robins, L. (eds) (1990) *Public Policy under Thatcher*, Basingstoke: Macmillan.

Scambler, A. and Scambler, G. (1981) 'Kinship and friendship networks and women's demand for primary care', *Journal, Royal College of General Practitioners* 26: 746–50.

Scambler, G. (1989) *Epilepsy*, London: Routledge.

Scambler, G. (ed.) (1991) *Sociology as Applied to Medicine*, London: Baillière Tindall.

Scott, R.A. (1972) 'A proposed framework for analysing deviance as a property of social order', in R.A. Scott and J.D. Douglas (eds) *Theoretical Perspectives on Deviance*, New York: Basic Books.

Scull, A. (1992) 'The social control of the mad', in A. Giddens (ed.) *Human*

Societies, Cambridge: Polity.

Scully, D. and Bart, P. (1978) 'A funny thing happened on the way to the orifice: the depiction of women in gynaecology textbooks', in J. Ehreinreich (ed.) *The Cultural Crisis of Modern Medicine*, New York: Monthly Review Press.

Sheppard, M. (1992) 'Contact and collaboration with general practitioners: a comparison of social workers and community nurses', *British Journal of Social Work* 22: 419–36.

Smith, D. (1989) *North and South*, London: Pelican.

Snaith, R. (ed.) (1989) *Neighbourhood Care and Social Policy*, London: HMSO.

St Leger, A.S., Schnieden, H. and Walsworth-Bell, J.P. (1992) *Evaluating Health Services' Effectiveness*, Milton Keynes: Open University Press.

Stacey, M. (1988) *The Sociology of Health and Healing*, London: Routledge.

Stainton Rogers, W. (1991) *Explaining Health and Illness*, London: Harvester Wheatsheaf.

Stern, J. (1983) 'Social mobility and the interpretation of social class mortality differentials', *Journal of Social Policy* 12, 1: 27–49.

Stewart, M. and Roter, D. (1989) *Communicating with Medical Patients*, New York: Sage Publications.

Strong, P. and Robinson, J. (1990) *The NHS – Under New Management*, Milton Keynes: Open University Press.

Szasz, T. (1975) *The Age of Madness: History of Involuntary Mental Hospitalisation*, London: Routledge & Kegan Paul.

Szasz, T. and Hollender, M.H. (1956) 'A contribution to the philosophy of medicine', *AMA Archives of Internal Medicine* XCVII: 585–92.

Titmuss, R. (1963) *Essays on the Welfare State*, London: George Allen & Unwin.

Townsend, P., Davidson, N. and Whitehead, M. (1988a) *Inequalities in Health*, London: Penguin.

Townsend, P., Phillimore, P. and Beattie, A. (1988b) *Health and Deprivation: Inequality and the North*, London: Croom Helm.

Tuckett, D. (1982) *Introduction to Medical Sociology*, London: Tavistock.

Tuckett, D., Boulton, M., Olsen, C. and Williams, A. (1985) *Meetings Between Experts: An Approach to Sharing Ideas in Medical Consultations*, London: Tavistock Publications.

Tudor Hart, J. (1971) 'The inverse care law' *Lancet* 1: 405–12.

Ungerson, C. (1987) *Policy is Personal*, London: Tavistock.

United Kingdom Central Council for Nursing, Midwifery and Health Visiting (UKCC) (1984) *Code of Professional Conduct for the Nurse, Midwife and Health Visitor*, London: UKCC.

Waddington, I. (1973) 'The role of hospitals in the development of modern medicine', *Sociology* 7: 211–24.

Wadsworth, M., Butterfield, W. and Blaney, R. (1971) *Health and Sickness: The Choice of Treatment*, London: Tavistock.

Walker, A. (1982) *Community Care*, Oxford: Robertson.

Weber, M. (1978) *Economy and Society: An Outline of Interpretive Sociology*, Berkeley: University of California Press.

West, C. (1992) 'A general manager's view of contemporary nursing issues', in J. Robinson, A. Gray and R. Elkan (eds) *Policy Issues in Nursing*, Milton Keynes: Open University Press.

Western, W.W. and Brown, J.B. (1989) 'The importance of patients' beliefs', in M. Stewart and D. Roter (eds) *Communicating with Medical Patients*, London: Sage.

Whitehead, M. (1987) *The Health Divide: Inequalities in Health in the 1980s*, London: Health Education Council.

Whitehead, M. (1988) 'The health divide', in P. Townsend, N. Davidson and M. Whitehead (eds) *Inequalities in Health*, London: Penguin.

Whitehead, M. (1992), 'The concepts and principles of equity and health', *International Journal of Health Services* 22, 3: 429–45

Whitehead, M. (1994) 'Who cares about equity in the NHS?' *British Medical Journal* 308: 1284–7.

Wilkinson, R. (1986) 'Income and mortality', in R. Wilkinson (ed.) *Class and Health: Research and Longitudinal Data*, London: Tavistock.

Williams, A. (1985) 'Economics of coronary artery bypass grafting', *British Medical Journal* 291, 6490: 328.

Williams, S. (1987) 'Goffman, interactionism, and the management of stigma in everyday life', in G. Scambler (ed.) *Sociological Theory and Medical Sociology*, London: Tavistock.

Wilson, A. (1985) *Family*, London: Tavistock.

Wistow, G., Hardy, B. and Leedham, I. (1993) 'Planning blight', *Health Service Journal* 103, 5340: 22–4.

Wistow, G., Knapp, M., Hardy, B. and Allen, C. (1992) 'From providing to enabling: local authorities and the mixed economy of social care', *Public Administration* 70: 25–45.

Wolfensberger, W. (1972) *The Principle of Normalisation in Human Services*, Toronto: National Institute of Mental Retardation.

Zola, I. (1973) 'Pathways to the doctor', *Social Science and Medicine* 7: 677-89.

Author index

Subject index

Entries in **bold type** indicate a key concept or term and a page number in bold type directs the reader to the page on which the meaning or definition of the concept or term appears.

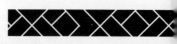